FOOD AND NUTRITION

WHAT EVERYONE NEEDS TO KNOW®

FOOD AND NUTRITION

WHAT EVERYONE NEEDS TO KNOW®

P.K. NEWBY, ScD, MPH, MS

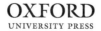
OXFORD
UNIVERSITY PRESS

OXFORD

UNIVERSITY PRESS

Oxford University Press is a department of the University of Oxford. It furthers
the University's objective of excellence in research, scholarship, and education
by publishing worldwide. Oxford is a registered trade mark of Oxford University
Press in the UK and certain other countries.

"What Everyone Needs to Know" is a registered trademark of
Oxford University Press.

Published in the United States of America by Oxford University Press
198 Madison Avenue, New York, NY 10016, United States of America.

© Oxford University Press 2018

Library of Congress Cataloging-in-Publication Data
Names: Newby, P.K., author.
Title: Food and nutrition : what everyone needs to know / P.K. Newby.
Description: New York, NY : Oxford University Press, [2018] |
Series: What everyone needs to know |
Includes bibliographical references and index.
Identifiers: LCCN 2018013010 (print) | LCCN 2018015508 (ebook) |
ISBN 9780190846657 (Updf) | ISBN 9780190846664 (Epub) |
ISBN 9780190846633 (paperback) | ISBN 9780190846640 (hardcover)
Subjects: LCSH: Nutrition—Popular works. | Food—Popular works. |
Health—Popular works. | BISAC: MEDICAL / General. | COOKING / General.
Classification: LCC RA784 (ebook) | LCC RA784 .N482 2018 (print) |
DDC 613.2—dc23
LC record available at https://lccn.loc.gov/2018013010

1 3 5 7 9 8 6 4 2

Paperback printed by Sheridan Books, Inc., United States of America
Hardback printed by Bridgeport National Bindery, Inc., United States of America

When you get right down to it,
food is practically the whole story every time.

—*Kurt Vonnegut*, Galápagos

CONTENTS

Part II Dining Throughout Human History: Science, Technology, Eater, Environment

3 How Revolutions, Discoveries, and Inventions Shape Our Diet: Paleo to Present   45

4 Contemporary Food Production, Buzzwords, and Pop Nutrition: Fact or Fiction?   56

7 Small and Mighty: Vitamins, Minerals, and Phytonutrients 109

8 The Foundation of Nutrition: Carbohydrate, Fat, and Protein 117

PREFACE: WHY IS NUTRITION CONFUSING, AND WHAT CAN BE DONE ABOUT IT?

Are you sometimes confused about what to eat for health? Do you want science-based information but don't know what to believe? Do you feel like nutritionists are always changing their minds? If so, you're not alone. And it's exactly why I wrote this book.

Its subtitle—*What Everyone Needs to Know* (and that means *you*)—is nonetheless a bit overwhelming and deeply humbling for this writer, for how can any single work cover the entirety of food and nutrition? After all, "[w]hen you get right down to it, food is practically the whole story every time" (in the wise words of American author Kurt Vonnegut). Thus, no individual book could ever do justice to this vast subject, covering in depth the myriad ways food shapes and impacts our health, environment, economy, and society. I try, even so, to provide what everyone needs to know, taking you on a journey that spans time, space, and place—and large bodies of literature across scientific disciplines like nutrition, agriculture, biology, and anthropology—to better understand how and why what we eat matters, from farm to fork.

But we live in a time of short attention spans fomented by fast-moving newsfeeds that never stop, and contemporary food and nutrition conversations are dominated by anti-science coming from all directions, including self-appointed gurus, Hollywood celebrities, well-meaning bloggers, snake oil salespeople, physicians with next to no training in nutrition—and your mother. People are hungrier than ever for evidence-based answers, but the din of junk science diet advice is deafening, fueling the oft-heard mantra, "Why is nutrition so confusing?"

The reality is that nutrition is rooted in biochemistry, and knowledge evolves over time, inching forward slowly, a science like any other. Even so, there is far more consensus about diet and health than you would believe: *a staggering 80% of chronic diseases are preventable through modifiable lifestyle changes such as diet*, which is the single largest contributing factor responsible for today's chronic disease pandemic. Moreover, modern food production is responsible for grave environmental damage to our land, water, and air and a major contributor to climate change. For these reasons and others, some believe we are undergoing a food revolution. Indeed, more and more people are taking a harder look at what's on their plate and how it got there—and demanding change in our food system. And I have hope that, decades from now, the tide on chronic disease will have ebbed and agriculture will have embraced more sustainable practices that protect eaters, farmworkers, and our beautiful planet Earth.

You may stumble across information in this book that does not concur with your current views. In these cases, I challenge you to question the source and basis of your information, open your mind, and perhaps follow the advice of Yoda, the sage Jedi master in *Star Wars*: "You must unlearn what you have learned." Indeed, the great futurist Alvin Toffler's similar words ring truer than ever in today's social media society that shrouds opinions as fact: "The illiterate of the 21st century will not be those who cannot read and write, but those who cannot learn, unlearn, and relearn." Science is not a belief system built on faith and unknowable truths but a systematic method of inquiry that, over time, creates a rich body of information illuminating the way the world works—and science is true whether you believe it or not, to paraphrase Neil deGrasse Tyson. In the case of nutrition science, this knowledge can literally save your own life—and maybe even the planet—and make the world a better, safer place for all creatures, great and small.

My ultimate goal is therefore that this book not only answers some of today's most pressing questions in a way that stimulates your mind but also leads to action. Perhaps it will whet your appetite for more information, and I encourage you to seek more detailed accounts of the science and history if you're so inclined. (A selected bibliography is provided at the book's end, and a complete list of the 1200+ references is found at pknewby.com.) Although this book is rooted in human health and disease, the realm of traditional nutrition, I also raise awareness about our culinary past and highlight critical issues in our present that encourage a more global and compassionate view of why food's influence lies far, far beyond our own bodies. While the book concludes by considering what tomorrow's supper will look like based on current trends in science and technology, paramount is the knowledge that it is we, everyday eaters, who shape the future of food with every choice we make, every bite we eat. Together, we possess the collective power to create the change in the world we wish to see, stimulating the necessary revolution we need to save ourselves and our planet.

P.K. Newby, ScD, MPH, MS

ACKNOWLEDGMENTS

This book would never have been written had I not had the good fortune (and good sense) to enroll in "Nutritional Ecology." It was the early 1990s, and Joan Gussow, EdD, led this class at Columbia University's Teacher's College. I was a new graduate student and quaffed hungrily every bit of knowledge I could about food and nutrition. The "Aha!" moment this course provided indelibly changed my life—and the course of my career. I jumped on the bandwagon, (still) proselytizing my own mantra "From farm to fork, what we eat matters!" and encouraging Harvard and other places to add environmental nutrition to their curriculum, with varying degrees of success. It is because of Dr. Gussow that "farm to fork" eating—nutrition ecology—became the organizing philosophy for the many courses I developed and taught over the years, helping students connect their dietary choices with impacts on the environment, economy, and society, not just personal health. The concepts are far from novel, yet remain eye opening, and life changing, to so many. Today's escalating climate change crisis has once again raised attention to how conventional agriculture is contributing to the destruction of our planet, and more and more eaters are taking a harder look at what's on their plate, and how it got there. I am deeply grateful to the countless students who have attended my classes over the years, and to the public as well, all of whom have come to hear me speak passionately about these issues—especially for their ongoing inspiration, intelligent questions, and warm support. I'm also very appreciative to Oxford University Press for publishing this necessary book, the first of its kind, with special thanks going to my editor, Angela Chnapko, for her patience and guidance throughout the process. Dr. Gregory Newby, my older brother, has been particularly supportive of my intellectual pursuits since the beginning and has been a wonderful mentor, sounding board, and editor from this book's conception. My dad, Neville Newby, gets a shout-out for being a life-long valued guide and friend, in all things, and my deep passion for food (gardening, cooking, baking, and the like) was cultivated as a child and is attributed solely to my mother, Linda Newby. My husband, Dr. Vilas Sridharan has been an ongoing source of support, emotionally and financially. And K'Ehleyr, our feisty black lab, has been my trusty writing companion, contributing to a peaceful environment (and also dragging me away from my desk for afternoon walks). I lastly and mostly thank you, the reader. Know that I'm with you every day as we strive toward better health, together. Here's to you!

FOOD AND NUTRITION

WHAT EVERYONE NEEDS TO KNOW®

Part I

WHY WHAT WE EAT MATTERS

FARM TO FORK

Our food supply is more plentiful than ever, yet many of the challenges we've faced throughout history, like famine, nutrient deficiencies, and hunger, still plague our world. And a range of new health conditions and chronic diseases has emerged as a function of longer lives and changing lifestyles. At the same time, grave environmental damages related to food production threaten our Earth, its people, and future generations. Who is responsible, and what is the path forward?

1

FRAMING TODAY'S FOOD AND NUTRITION ISSUES

What's this book about?

The *Oxford Living Dictionary* defines "food" as "a nutritious substance that people or animals eat or drink or that plants absorb in order to maintain life and growth." It cites the often-used phrase "food for thought" as "Something that warrants serious consideration." Both are perfect fodder to begin this book.

The contents herein focus on food in the literal sense, including the who, what, where, when, how, and why surrounding the basic act of eating. The goal is to provide, as the title suggests, everything you need to know when it comes to food and nutrition. At the book's core is the question: how does what we eat impact health, longevity, and disease? An additional goal is to demonstrate how contemporary diet trends, whether gluten-free or Paleo-only, can be viewed through a scientific lens; this allows readers to understand whether such fads are meaningful for health or just plain hooey. How food choices are made and the way in which our eating environments shape our diets are also part of "what everyone needs to know" as it's this information that steers and empowers the lasting and meaningful behavior change—yes, it is possible!—that enables healthy living.

Yet as important as physical nourishment is the food for thought this book offers. Indeed, "when you get right down to it, food is practically the whole story every time," wrote author Kurt Vonnegut in his novel *Galápagos*. Thus, an additional aim is to expand the lens through which you view supper throughout time, space, and place.

Far more than a delivery vehicle for powerful nutrients fundamental to human life—and the foundation of health—food is a source of pleasure, a celebration of culture, the very cornerstone of the development of civilization itself. And our diet affects more than just our own lives, as each bite shapes the larger food system, society, and environment when considered on a global scale. Who grew that food, and were farmers fairly compensated? What natural and synthetic resources were used? How does food production impact our shared planet's land, air, and water? And is food indeed a fundamental human right, as asserted by the Food and Agriculture Organization of the United Nations (FAO)? The right to food was first noted in the Universal Declaration of Human Rights of the United Nations in 1948, noting "hunger is both a violation of human dignity and an obstacle to social, political and economic progress." The rights framework was further specified in 1999 as "when every man, woman, and child, alone or in community with others, has the physical and economic access at all times to adequate food or means for its procurement." (FAO works directly with governments and nonprofit organizations to implement "right to food" guidelines.) Whether you consciously consider such issues during mealtime or not, the fact nonetheless remains that diet doesn't just impact our health or the environment: how and what we eat reflect our personal values and ethics, a vote for the kind of food system we want. As a society, what we eat matters, from farm to fork.

May this book afford an opportunity to consider your own relationship with food and to arm yourself with evidence-based information so that you might create a healthier today for yourself—and a more sustainable tomorrow for the Earth. There is no "one size fits all" when it comes to diet, and these goals can be achieved harmoniously in a way that suits your palate, preference, and lifestyle.

Who should read this book? Is a science background necessary?

As its subtitle states, this book is for everyone. That means *you*. Its major aim is to provide an overview of what you need to know in order to harness the power of nutrition to foster health, prevent disease, and live longer. While popular nutrition and food topics are included, so is a crash course in nutrition, to provide the necessary lens to view current controversies and understand contemporary food conversations. That's because you need some background in the basics—particularly how fats, carbs, and proteins impact the body—in order to sort fact from fiction. But no previous background is necessary as you'll get what you need right here. Helping you become science-savvy about nutrition is a key goal of the book since newsfeeds are never-ending, abounding with anti-science that undermines your ability to make sound choices. This book will arm you with the information you need to "just say no" to junk science.

To that end, this book is evidence-based, meaning the information comes mainly from scientific studies published in peer-reviewed journals. Consensus reports from international nongovernmental organizations like the World Health Organization (WHO) and FAO are drawn from broadly, as are reports from scientific agencies in the US and Europe, England in particular. High-quality articles from the popular press are also referenced—there are many terrific sources!—as this is the place where most eaters get their information. At the end of the book you'll find a list of selected readings referenced herein, which is only a small portion; the complete bibliography may be found at pknewby.com. A list of acronyms commonly used in this book follows:

- BMI—body mass index
- CAFO—concentrated animal feeding operation
- CDC—Centers for Disease Control and Prevention
- CHD—coronary heart disease
- CVD—cardiovascular disease
- DHA—docasahexaenoic acid (an omega-3 fat)
- DNA—deoxyribonucleic acid
- EFSA—European Food Safety Authority
- EPA—US Environmental Protection Agency
- EPA—eicosapentaenoic acid (an omega-3 fat)
- EU—European Union
- FAO—Food and Agriculture Organization of the United Nations
- FDA—US Food & Drug Administration
- GE—genetic engineering/genetically engineered

- GHG—greenhouse gas
- GHGe—greenhouse gas emission
- GMO—genetically modified organism
- HDL—high-density lipoprotein ("good") cholesterol
- LDL—low-density lipoprotein ("bad") cholesterol
- MUFA—monounsaturated fatty acid (aka, monounsaturated fat)
- PUFA—polyunsaturated fatty acid (aka, polyunsaturated fat)
- RCT—randomized controlled trial
- RNA—ribonucleic acid
- SFA—saturated fatty acid (aka, saturated fat)
- T2DM—type 2 diabetes mellitus
- UK—United Kingdom
- UN—United Nations
- US—United States
- USDA—US Department of Agriculture
- WHO—World Health Organization
- WWF—World Wildlife Fund

In addition, abbreviations used in metric measurement (mg for milligram, m for meter, mL for liter, and the like) are employed throughout, and colloquial shorthand in nutrition is also commonly used (e.g., "sat fat" for saturated fat, "carbs" for carbohydrates).

While the results from individual experiments are sometimes included, particularly if research in an area is scarce or a specific study is especially exciting, I most often refer to investigations that have examined the results of an entire body of literature. Such studies may take the form of a systematic review, Cochrane review, or meta-analysis, all of which utilize specific statistical methods and criteria to evaluate the overall strength of the evidence across many, many studies (e.g., are high-protein diets better for weight loss than high-carb diets?) and often include tens or hundreds of thousands of people—and sometimes even millions. Relying on sources like these is imperative as one study, however intriguing, must be reproduced, its results corroborated by additional experiments in diverse settings, before findings can be considered facts. This is a slow process; that is how science works. While some studies may make for interesting news, results touted as truth by the media often lack context, contributing to confusion about what to eat. A prime example is the hyperbolic headlines usually based on individual experiments, a phenomenon I refer to as "single study sensationalism." My hope is that this book will help you avoid falling prey to the constant clickbait our culture has created.

And, unlike celebrity nutrition based on little more than anecdote, this book relies upon scientific disciplines like nutritional epidemiology, which examines how diet impacts health and disease in different populations. Epidemiology uses statistics to measure how a given dietary "exposure" (e.g., walnuts, kale, beef) is related to a specific health "outcome," or disease (e.g., heart disease, obesity, cancer). Epidemiologic studies are "observational," meaning data are collected from people like you going about their lives, eating the way they eat, losing and gaining weight, and so forth. Some are better than others: prospective studies that follow people over time are best as they ensure that the association was because the exposure preceded the disease and wasn't simply correlated. You are likely familiar with the phrase "correlation does not equal causation," and that axiom is fundamental when thinking about diet and disease.

Randomized controlled trials (RCTs, aka intervention studies or clinical trials) are a critical part of the picture since assigning some people to eat certain foods while others do not (who form the placebo, or control, group) is part of how we can ensure the dietary element in question was the salient factor. All that said, no study design is perfect, which is why we rely upon a great many to reproduce the results. And we often draw upon data from animal studies and laboratory (in vitro) experiments to understand not only what is happening but why, which is the "mechanism" of the disease. Only when the evidence converges from all sources do we reach consensus that a particular thing "causes" something else.

In nutritional epidemiology, statistics are used to measure associations between diet and disease and provide an estimate of risk, or odds, which are then presented as percentages (e.g., those consuming 5 servings of nuts weekly had an $x\%$ lower risk of heart disease compared to those who consumed less than 1 serving). Risk is always "relative" to something else and generally expressed with a degree of 95% certainty. To keep the text moving along, I refer simply to the magnitude of risk; interested readers may consult the studies themselves for more details.

Finally, while this book is designed to provide "what everyone needs to know" to build a health-promoting, disease-preventing, and life-giving diet, it is not possible for one book alone to provide "everything you need to know." While the material herein is applicable to pretty much everyone, some may have specific health conditions or diseases that alter nutritional needs. Or your genetic background or other lifestyle factors may carry specific risks that, together with this book, can be used to fine-tune your diet for optimal health. But don't lose the forest for the trees: 80% of chronic diseases can be prevented through lifestyle choices like diet—and the fundamentals you need are within these pages.

How do traditional and contemporary diets differ around the world?

Traditional food patterns are often defined by FAO as staple foods, those "eaten regularly and in such quantities as to constitute the dominant part of the diet and supply a major proportion of energy and nutrient needs." Traditional food practices arose from agriculture's humble beginnings (Chapter 3), a result of what the climate offered, in season, as a function of air temperature and humidity, soil quality, and proximity to water (notably, the coastline). Celebration, season, culture, and religious beliefs also shape traditional eating behaviors. Hindus, for example, do not eat beef, while Muslims do not consume pork.

Cereal grasses were among the first crops cultivated during the agricultural revolution (Chapter 3) and include sorghum (Africa), rice (China), maize (Central/South America), and wheat (Middle/ Near East). These four grains still characterize traditional diets and remain a staple of contemporary meals around the world; oats, rye, barley, and millet also contribute and vary globally according to regional growing conditions. Rice paddies predominate in lowland tropical environments and prevail in South and Southeast Asia. Maize (corn) can grow in tropical as well as temperate areas and is common in South and East Africa as well as Central America.

Africa's large semi-arid Sahelian region (including western and north-central Africa) favors millet and sorghum. Wheat is suited to temperate environments and is common in some regions of Europe and Central Asia—but absent in sub-Saharan Africa. Places with diverse geographic conditions produce several cereal crops, like wheat and maize in both North and South America. Still today, cereal grains contribute more than half of the world's total daily energy intake (i.e., calories). Rice, wheat, and maize alone contribute approximately 60% to energy intake worldwide and are vital protein sources in cultures where animal consumption is limited.

Vegetables further characterize traditional diets, predominantly roots and tubers but also leafy greens; species varies by climate. Beans, legumes, and nuts are part of many traditional diets around the world, including Central America and Africa in particular as well as North America—though the type of bean varies (Chapter 11). Peanuts are prominent in traditional African cuisine, for instance, while soybeans reign supreme in Asian diets. Traditional crops still characterize diets across the world, whether coffee, okra, and palm oil in Africa; bamboo, tea, and peach in China; eggplant, chickpea, and mango in South Asia; squash and sweet potato in Central and South America; or fig, pistachio, and almond in the Near East. Fruits contribute to global diets to a smaller degree due to their narrower growing season (and relatively low calorie content, perhaps); they are also expensive relative to other foods. Herbs and spices give traditional diets their flair, again related to the environment that originally provided them naturally prior to cultivation. Interestingly, of the estimated 400 000 plant species on Earth, at least half of which are likely edible for humans, only a tiny fraction are regularly consumed both traditionally and still today. While difficult to quantify, a 2007 analysis using FAO data (based on food weight, calories, protein, and fat) estimates that only about 25 foods comprise 90% of the world's diet (Table 1.1).

Like plants, the contribution of animal foods and products to traditional diets is also dictated by geography. Fish and seafood only characterized meals in coastal areas and those near freshwaters. These foods thus became a part of both traditional Mediterranean (e.g., Greece, Spain, and Italy) and Nordic (Denmark, Finland, Iceland, Norway, and Sweden) diets, for example. While both include an array of grains and vegetables, Nordic diets feature oats,

Table 1.1 25 Crops/Species Contribute 90% of Diet Intake Worldwide[a]

Apple
Banana and plantain
Bean
Barley
Cassava
Coconut
Grape
Groundnuts
Maize
Millet
Olive oil
Onion
Orange and mandarin
Palm oil
Potato
Rape and mustard oils
Rice
Sorghum
Soybean
Sugar cane
Sunflower oil
Sweet potato
Tomato
Wheat
Alcoholic and fermented beverages

[a]List also includes fruits, other; oils, other; pulses, other; sweeteners, other; and vegetables, other. (Notation reflects FAO convention.)

rye, cruciferous vegetables, native berries, and rapeseed oil, while the warmer Mediterranean diet boasts a wider array of vegetables and fruits, olive oil, and wheat. Both diets include seafood like salmon; there are different salmon species indigenous to each region.

Though relatively few in numbers, the Arctic-dwelling Inuit is a notable exception to the world's many traditional diets that are otherwise plant-based. The frigid climate is unsuitable for cultivating crops; hence, a food culture arose based on hunting, fishing, and gathering that includes sea mammals (like whale and seal), land mammals (like caribou), and birds. Animals (meat, dairy, eggs, and the like) gradually became a part of many other traditional diets to a small degree, especially goats and their milk. (Goat remains the most commonly consumed animal globally, Chapter 12.) Animal foods provide essential nutrients on family farms, particularly for subsistence farmers in the developing world.

Elements of traditional diets remain in many regions around the world, especially in rural and remote regions of low- and middle-income nations where infrastructure, income, and policies are prohibitive and diets are limited to foods locally available—and affordable. A major difference is the quantity of animal products consumed. In western Europe, for instance, 33% of energy intake on average comes from animal products compared to cereals (26%) and roots and tubers (4%). In contrast, cereals are the largest contributor to African diets on average (46%) compared to roots and tubers (20%) and animal products (7%). Meat and dairy are a hallmark of contemporary diets, a historical marker of wealth that still resonates today; and consumption is increasing alongside growing incomes, particularly in China.

Over time, humans learned to press oils from a wide range of crops, like palm, soy, and olive, gradually incorporating them to a small degree into traditional diets. (The cost to produce them was greater than consuming the plants whole.) Sugar was likewise cultivated and used in confections that varied culturally, though it contributed only when technology allowed (Chapter 4). And alcohol made from local crops, including rice (sake) or millet (brandy) in Asia and grapes (wine) in the Mediterranean, also contributed moderately to some traditional diets.

Traditional food and drink habits were diluted over time when invading cultures brought their own plants, animals, and food traditions to new lands, whether forcibly or through trade. Tea came to India by way of the British Empire, for example, which before then arrived in England from China via the Silk Road. Centuries-old influences like these can shape how "traditional" diet patterns are conceived. A traditional Latin American diet, for example, is often characterized not only by the indigenous diets of native Aztec, Incan, and Mayan cultures but also by more recent Spanish, Portuguese, and African influences.

In more recent history, improvements in food processing (Chapter 4) and quicker transportation have created a global food system, enabling food habits independent of season or tradition. The later decades of the 20th century hence saw the increasing prevalence of the so-called Western diet pattern, characterized by highly processed and refined food and beverages rich in sugar, sodium, and calories and high intakes of meat, dairy, and fast food. Fizzy drinks and fast food are hallmarks of Western diets. Coca-Cola (which means "delicious happiness" in Mandarin, according to the company's website) manufacturing began in 1886, and 1.9 billion people today enjoy Coca-Cola beverages daily across 200+ countries. And McDonald's is the largest food franchise globally, present in 36 000 locations across 100+ countries. Thus, some of the unique local customs and practices that once defined traditional diets around the world have been crowded out as globalization, acculturation, and urbanization have made westernized food culture pervasive. These dietary changes pose risks to both human and environmental health—and threaten the existence of age-old vibrant food cultures.

Who runs the food system?

FAO defines a food system as that which "embraces all the elements (environment, people, inputs, processes, infrastructure, institutions, markets, and trade) and activities that relate to the production, processing, distribution and marketing, preparation and consumption of food and the outputs of these activities, including socioeconomic and environmental outcomes." It further defines a sustainable food system as one that fosters food and nutrition security across economic, social, and environmental dimensions without compromising the needs of future generations.

The environmental impacts associated with a given food throughout the system are often measured using the life cycle assessment (LCA) process—namely, production, harvesting, post-harvesting, processing, retail, consumption, and waste disposal, as well as associated transportation costs. LCA quantifies the energy cost of resources used and greenhouse gases (GHGs) emitted at each step, including fuel costs associated with machinery and transport as well as raw materials like fertilizers, pesticides, and water; it thus enables comparisons that inform sustainability efforts (e.g., organic versus conventional systems, Chapter 4). The social and economic impacts of food choices start with production: who is growing food, and under what conditions? Agriculture has played a major role in development and was the main livelihood around the world for centuries. The services sector surpassed agriculture in 2000, a function of fewer jobs in farming and increasing wealth and opportunities elsewhere. While 1 in 3 people worldwide are still employed in agriculture in some way—most often by necessity, not choice—two-thirds of these are in low- and middle-income nations compared to 4% in high-income countries (Table 1.2). Variability exists: around 60% of the labor force works in agriculture in sub-Saharan Africa and 75% in Madagascar, compared to only about 1% in the United Kingdom (UK) and the United States (US). Agriculture is still growing in the developing world, particularly in South Asia and sub-Saharan Africa. Almost 80% of the world's harvested croplands are in low- and middle-income countries, and the net area harvested across 140 developing nations grew by 14% between 2000 and 2010; 12 countries—8 in Africa alone—saw an astonishing increase of 50% or more.

A 2014 FAO report on the state of food and agriculture estimated that 90% of the world's 570 million farms were managed by families, which produce about 80% of the world's food and draw upon about 75% of all agricultural resources. The majority of family farms (84%) are less than 2 hectares in size. Yet farms greater than 50 hectares

Table 1.2 Where Are the World's Farms?[a]

China—35%

India—24%

Rest of Asia—15%

Sub-Saharan Africa—9%

Europe & Central Asia—7%

Latin America & Caribbean—4%

High-income countries—4%

Middle East & North Africa—3%

[a]Data are from FAO, 2014.

(1%), many of which are family-managed, control 65% of all agricultural land. The bulk of these large farms are located in middle- and high-income countries, many of which are dedicated to livestock. The two largest farms in the world are in China, a gargantuan 22 500 000 acres and 11 000 000 acres, both dairy farms that house 100 000 and 40 000 cows, respectively.

Agriculture is currently declining in regions with growing wealth, like East Asia, Latin America, and the Caribbean, just as it has in the US, the UK, and other high-income nations. In the US, 1.4% of Americans (2.6 million) are operating some 2.1 million farms, producing fuel and fiber as well as food; 99% of farms remain family-owned, though they are far larger in acreage today on average than in previous decades. Around 75% of agricultural sales are under $50 000, with 57% under $10 000, the latter of which comprises only 1% of production. Farmers are becoming older on average, and fewer each year enter the industry: there was an approximately 20% drop in the number of new (principal) farmers from 2007 to 2012. Further, farming is not a full-time job for many American farmers today: 62% spend days working off the farm, and 52% have a primary occupation other than farming.

While farming used to be a stand-alone industry, various points of the production chain became more interconnected throughout the 20th century, leading to the coined portmanteau "agribusiness" in 1957. While the term simply refers to the business of a range of food production activities, agribusiness is often used pejoratively in connection with "Big Food"— that is, the multinational food and beverage industry with huge and concentrated market power—to underscore its wide reach across so many aspects of the food system. Big Food examples include global powerhouses Nestlé, Anheuser-Busch InBev, and Coca-Cola, the three biggest publicly traded food and beverage companies in the world in 2016, which produce far more than the respective chocolate, beer, and soda their names suggest. Nestlé (est. 1866), for instance, boasts more than 2000 brands that run the culinary gamut—chocolate, candy, dairy, baby food, coffee, pet food, frozen food, beverages, and so forth—reflecting a long history of mergers and acquisitions. In 2013, the "Big Six" multinationals (which became the "Big Four" in 2017) controlled 75% of the agrochemical market and 63% of the commercial seed market, raising questions about monopolistic control furthering the use of agrochemicals in food production and increasing prices for farmers.

Still, there is not a single food system. Alternative food systems (e.g., organic) arise and grow even among the Big Food players to address escalating concerns about the social, environmental, and economic sustainability of conventional methods. And local and regional systems continue to play an essential role in feeding people in the developing world, where time-honored and novel production methods are employed to meet food needs. Many are engaged in subsistence farming, producing food only for household consumption (not trade or sale), or are small shareholders. In fact, only 12% of harvested croplands in the developing world produce cash crops (e.g., sugar, coffee, cocoa, palm oil, tea), many of which are exported to wealthier nations.

Big or small, global or local, *all* food systems must become more sustainable to ensure food and nutrition security for future generations, a dynamic process that varies greatly with people and place.

Who produces and provides our food?

Worldwide, more women than men participate in agriculture (around 38% versus 33% on average), with 70% female workers in South Asia and 60% in sub-Saharan Africa. Yet there remains a significant gender gap: women in agriculture are provided fewer assets, inputs, services, technologies, and extension and financial services as well as less land, livestock, education, and labor, all of which reduce unnecessarily their productivity. Indeed, many women work without any pay at all, unable to manage even their own time. On average, women own only 30% of land globally. Numerous studies indicate that increasing support for women in farming, in all ways, supports families and local economies. Paramount is increasing the status and power of women in the household, and ensuring rights to manage both income and time is essential. An analogous situation exists in fishing and fish farming: women play a critical role—making up half the workforce in inland fisheries, for example—but are often uncounted and lack the same rights or recognitions as male fishers.

Children are also major participants in agriculture, which employs more young people than any other industry worldwide. An estimated 152 million children, half of whom reside in Africa, worked in farming, livestock, forestry, fishing, or aquaculture in 2017; 108 million of them were between 5 and 17 years of age. Many children are forced to leave school to participate in often dangerous agricultural activities to provide labor for impoverished farming families.

Although most child labor occurs in sugar cane and coffee production, the cocoa industry is also a major perpetrator. An estimated 70% of cocoa comes from two countries in West Africa, Côte d'Ivoire and Ghana. Cocoa farmers are often unable to negotiate fair wages due to concentrated control within the industry, and this creates the demand for child labor. While most child laborers work for their families, others enter the workforce as a result of child trafficking and slavery. Although increased media attention has led to some industry improvements—and slow progress is being made—an estimated 2.1 million children were still involved in the chocolate industry in West Africa in 2016, where farm wages still fall well below the international poverty line. And child labor has actually *increased* in recent years, likely due to growing demand for chocolate in places with growing disposable income, like India and China.

Human trafficking in general is another challenge facing agriculture. In 2016, an estimated 24.9 million people were forced to work with little or no pay, 11% of whom worked in agriculture and fishing. (This number is likely an underestimate due to the difficulty in accurately counting victims.) A wide variety of techniques are used in human trafficking to control workers, including violence and abuse, threats of deportation, lies, debt, and physical restraint. Forced labor happens ubiquitously, including in the US, where most are immigrants—the majority of whom are legal (about 70%).

One of the most egregious examples of modern slavery in US agriculture was among tomato farmworkers living in Immokalee, Florida. A small group began organizing in 1993 to address the cruel working conditions, which grew into the Coalition of Immokalee Workers (CIW). In its first 20 years, CIW helped detect and prosecute numerous cases of slavery, ultimately liberating more than 1200 workers. In 2015, the group turned its attention to tomato farms in Georgia, South Carolina, North Carolina, Maryland, Virginia, and

New Jersey; it also advocated for workers harvesting strawberries and peppers in Florida and producing dairy in Vermont. While the CIW illustration is extreme, farmworkers in general (often migrant or seasonal workers or immigrants) are considered among the most economically disadvantaged labor group in the US. CIW has since extended its reach further down the food system to the corporate food industry and retailers driving unfair wages (and, in some cases, forced labor and slavery) in order to keep prices low for consumers. Through boycotts and other methods, CIW obtained wage increases by reaching fair food agreements with businesses in the tomato supply chain, including big box stores like Walmart, supermarkets such as Whole Foods and Trader Joe's, and fast food chains including Taco Bell and McDonald's. The CIW example and others like it demonstrate the importance of considering not just the "who" of food production but also the "how"; that is, the practices employed throughout the supply chain, beginning with farmworkers.

What are the major food and nutrition challenges impacting human and environmental health?

Nutrition is a scientific discipline focused on understanding the impact of food and nutrients on health and disease (Part III). Nutritional problems (Chapter 2) generally relate to both the quantity and quality of food in the diet, ranging from insufficient energy intake (undernutrition) to intake imbalanced with expenditure (overnutrition). Inadequate consumption of nutrients required for health, growth, and development (malnutrition) mostly occurs as a consequence of limited food intake or reliance upon too few foods that constrains nutrient intake. Malnutrition may also occur in overnourished individuals if the diet is severely imbalanced.

For the vast majority of human history, humans were most likely to suffer from under- and malnutrition due to food scarcity. These remain major public health challenges across the globe, particularly in low- and middle-income countries. FAO defines undernourishment (aka, undernutrition) as an inability to acquire enough food to meet daily minimum dietary energy (calorie) requirements for normal health and activity during the course of a year; chronic undernourishment is defined as hunger. Hunger is not due to an insufficient food supply: the world produces more than enough calories to feed every person on the planet. Rather, hunger is the primary result of poverty, as well as sociopolitical factors that prevent access and distribution like natural disasters, wars and conflicts, financial crises impacting food price and trade, and inadequate infrastructure. During the later decades of the 20th century, some scientists became increasingly cognizant of food's impact not just on individual human bodies but also on our shared local and global environments. Thus emerged a discipline sometimes referred to as "nutritional ecology," or environmental nutrition. The four-quadrant model of nutritional ecology includes health, environment, economy, and society and is the working model for this book; it emphasizes health and environmental aspects of food choices in particular.

Of course, the idea that how we grow, produce, and distribute food impacts systems beyond our own health is not new. In 1906, Upton Sinclair's *The Jungle* highlighted atrocities in the American meatpacking industry, which mostly impacted the working poor, recent immigrants to the US. This seminal work led to the 1906 Pure Food and Drug Act and the Meat Inspection Act, which improved conditions and protected workers. More than 50 years later Rachel Carson's *Silent Spring* (1962) detailed the impact of agricultural chemicals on ecosystems and human health. It is credited for launching the modern environmental movement. The cry for a more sustainable food system and less meat consumption was the topic of Frances Moore Lappé's *Diet for a Small Planet* (1971). And philosopher Peter Singer's treatise *Animal Liberation: A New Ethics for Our Treatment of Animals* (1975) discouraged consumption of animals by decrying "speciesism," which challenges the notion that any one species owns another and argues that it is the ability to suffer—not intelligence—that should guide our treatment of animals and, hence, their consumption. More recently, Peter Singer and Jim Mason's *The Ethics of What We Eat* (2006) sounded a siren on the inhumane ways in which animals are raised for food production.

Many of the same environmental nutrition issues introduced in these books remain problems today; some have grown in magnitude, like water and land pollution. Still others, like antibiotic resistance (Chapter 12) and climate change (Chapter 2), are newly appreciated as mounting threats to local communities and the global environment.

How can we solve food and nutrition problems? Revolution, or evolution?

In many cases, the science and technology and evidence-based best practices already exist to address, ameliorate, and even eliminate the majority of today's global food and nutrition challenges. Potential solutions are situated philosophically and politically, a reflection of fundamental belief systems regarding the roles and responsibilities of government, society, and individuals in health and disease. Deep-seated values about science and nature are also pertinent to framing problems and solutions, particularly in the face of new technologies like genetic engineering (Chapters 3 and 4).

The field of public health employs the social–ecological model, which places the individual within a network of personal relationships (e.g., family, friends) and organizations (e.g., schools, workplaces, faith-based organizations) that are in turn shaped by public policy and societal influences. Thus, the individual is ultimately responsible for bringing fork to mouth but is nonetheless part of a larger system that influences food choices, eating behaviors, and hence health and disease. Consequently, there are myriad levels across which efforts to improve nutrition can occur, often with varying degrees of impact. Interventions directed toward few people that also require behavior modification are limited in scope and efficacy. Moreover, education alone does not often lead to behavior change in most cases. (Think, for example, of those who smoke, despite knowing its role in lung cancer.) Interventions in the food environment and health policy arenas that impact populations but require little or no individual effort, like food fortification programs and food safety regulations, are better poised to improve outcomes. Major health improvements are also seen when underlying socioeconomic issues are addressed that thwart healthful choices, like insufficient income or health insurance.

While scientists and professionals across a broad range of disciplines work to address global food and nutrition challenges, public awareness of and investment in food and nutrition issues play powerful roles in driving change. History repeats itself once again as a new generation of journalists and social activists flood light on a food system that continues to degrade the environment, escalate climate change, abuse farm animals, exploit agricultural workers, and harm human health. The role of nutrition in obesity and other chronic diseases is receiving greater media attention than ever before, as is the impact of food production and agricultural practices on the environment. Writers like Michael Pollan (*The Omnivore's Dilemma*, 2007), Eric Schlosser (*Fast Food Nation*, 2001), and Anna Lappé (who continues the work her mother began with *Diet for a Hot Planet: The Climate Crisis at the End of Your Fork and What You Can Do About It*, 2010) have inspired countless community groups, nonprofit organizations, and individuals to think critically about how they eat. Many chefs have also taken up various causes, including the No Child Hungry campaign. In 2010, England's celebrity chef Jamie Oliver even called for a "Food Revolution Day" focused on childhood obesity and school nutrition. The US later jumped on board with its own Food Day, launched in 2011 by the consumer organization Center for Science in the Public Interest. Long before these, World Food Day was established by FAO in 1979 to raise awareness about world hunger.

These are only a sample of the myriad activities surrounding food and nutrition, fueling what many see as a growing food revolution. There can be no question that all point to a mounting interest in how food is produced and how that food affects our health, longevity, and planet. But is there truly a "food revolution"? Perhaps not, if a revolution is defined sociologically as radical change that occurs rather quickly. Calls have been made for changes to the food system and protections for public health and the environment throughout modern history—and many of the same alarms still ring today.

Notably, many calling for "food revolution" come from places of privilege: those with time, energy, and resources to dedicate to such activities. Attention is often centered around what might be considered "first world food problems" (e.g., Is it "natural"? Or genetically engineered? And will it make me fat?). Yet literally billions continue to suffer from diseases that largely impact individuals of lower socioeconomic status and those living in low- and middle-income countries, problems like hunger, malnutrition, and shorter life spans that disproportionately affect women, children, and people of color. And these same individuals are also more likely to live in environments with greater land, water, and air pollution.

This is not to say that such questions are frivolous; they contribute to a growing conversation about why what we eat matters, farm to fork. It is nevertheless striking that there is so little public awareness of, or media attention to, ongoing food and nutrition tragedies that still pervade our world in astronomical proportions. And those facing such problems, daily, are unable to speak for themselves, suitably focused as they are on meeting their basic requirements of food, water, and safety—when possible.

Whether complex issues like hunger and health disparities will ever receive the public attention and outrage they warrant, or ever be the focal point of a "food revolution," seems uncertain. Only 15% of Americans were even aware of the four (near) famines in 2017 facing at least 20 million in South Sudan, Somalia, Nigeria, and Yemen, for example, what the International Rescue Committee called the "least reported but most important issue of our time." What is likely, however, is that, over time—centuries, millennia—today's major food and nutrition problems will be solved through the course of scientific discovery, technology, and innovation that are the hallmarks of human evolution.

2

GLOBAL FOOD AND NUTRITION CHALLENGES

PEOPLE AND PLANET

Who is affected by hunger, food insecurity, and malnutrition?

Global hunger has been decreasing steadily in recent years, from about 900 million in 2000 to 777 million in 2015, or about 1 in 9 individuals worldwide. Despite population growth, hunger in the developing world fell from 23.3% in 1990–1992 to 12.9% in 2015. Alas, hunger (or chronic malnourishment) and related conditions showed an uptick in 2016, impacting 816 million. Most affected are those in regions of sub-Saharan Africa, southeastern Asia, and western Asia, where conflict and violence, in combination with droughts or floods, have led to famines.[1] In February 2017, the United Nations (UN) declared a famine in South Sudan, the first official famine since 2011 and the most severe since World War II. An ongoing civil war—causing a "man-made famine"—has destroyed crops and markets and thwarted food aid. South Sudan (the world's newest country) is one of four nations, including Yemen, Nigeria, and Somalia, that faced war-related famine in 2017. In aggregate, some 20 million people were at risk of starvation due to food (and water) shortages. The Food and Agriculture Organization (FAO) 2017 report *"The State of Food Security and Nutrition in the World"* therefore called the nexus of conflict, food security, and nutrition an "imperative for sustainable peace."

Regions with the highest prevalence of hunger are sub-Saharan Africa and South Asia. Women are more likely than men to suffer from undernourishment, often due to gender discrimination and inadequate women's rights. Food insecurity—defined by the United States Department of Agriculture (USDA) Economic Research Service as homes without adequate food for all household members—is a related problem that results in acute rather than chronic malnourishment. Food insecurity is not just an issue in low- and middle-income nations: in the United States (US), 12.7% of households, or approximately 42.2 million Americans, were food-insecure in 2015. Individuals in low-income households or living in the South and those headed by single women or people of color, primarily black or Hispanic, had the lowest food security.

Hunger impacts health in numerous ways, and the International Food Policy Research Institute redefined it in 2015 to encompass three unique states: child wasting (low weight for height), reflecting acute undernutrition; child stunting (low height for age), reflecting chronic undernutrition; and child mortality, often reflecting critical nutrient deficiencies (malnutrition) alongside other environmental stressors like lack of safe drinking water. According to the World Food Programme, half of all deaths in children under 5 years old are due to undernutrition.

Malnutrition impacts billions globally, primarily women and children. It is sometimes referred to as "hidden hunger." The chief micronutrient deficiencies are iron, vitamin A, iodine, zinc, and folate. Iron deficiency anemia is most common and impacts some 33% of women of reproductive age globally and 2 billion people overall, particularly in the developing world; anemia results in ill health and lack of productivity among adults and 1 in 5 maternal deaths. Anemia due to folate deficiency is also common. Vitamin A deficiency affects 250 million children worldwide, and as many as 500 000 will become blind as a result; half of these will die if untreated. A lack of iodine in the diet is the largest contributor to preventable brain damage, and 54 countries remain iodine-deficient, although global prevalence has been cut in half over the past several decades. Approximately 1 in 3 worldwide have insufficient zinc intake, which increases risk of infections like malaria and diarrhea; sub-Saharan Africa, South Asia, and India have the highest prevalence. All of the aforementioned conditions are due to inadequate vitamin or mineral intake, but many also suffer from a lack of protein in the diet, resulting in kwashiorkor (protein-energy malnutrition).

Finally, around 1 billion people lack access to safe drinking water, and approximately 115 people die hourly—and 1 child every 15 seconds—from water-related diseases. Groundwater is increasingly scarce, which impacts as many as 4 billion today according to recent studies, a result of a severe drop in the water table related to both population growth and climate change. A January 2018 report from the World Resources Institute estimated that 33 countries around the world would face extreme water stress by 2040. And water shortages, like food shortages, are major causes of civil unrest that threaten peace as well as health, as seen in Iran in 2017.

What is obesity, and why is it a health problem?

While hunger and malnutrition have existed since the beginning of time, a relatively new nutritional problem faced by humans is overnutrition. Overnutrition is caused by an imbalance between energy intake and expenditure—calories in exceed calories out—that results in excess body fat relative to lean body mass. Overweight is generally measured using body mass index (BMI), an indirect ratio of fat mass relative to body weight (weight in kg divided by height in m squared), where a BMI of 25 to 30 reflects overweight and a BMI of 30 or above reflects obesity. Abdominal obesity, a function of excess waist circumference where fat accumulates in the central region of the body, is particularly harmful to cardiovascular health independent of BMI. During the 1980s, overnutrition began rising among adults in high-income nations, where food is plentiful, and the above BMI cutoff points were established due to their association with excess morbidity and mortality. (Cutoff points are used internationally and are a valid measure of overweight and obesity among the vast majority of people, with a few exceptions.) In the US today, more than 2 in 3 adults and 1 in 3 children are overweight or obese. And 35% of adult men and 40% of women and 17% of children aged 2–19 years were obese between 2011 and 2014.

Obesity is no longer relegated to high-income countries. Increasing industrialization and urbanization in tandem with changing diets and decreasing physical activity in the developing world have contributed to the growing prevalence of global obesity, which has more than doubled since 1980. Today, rising overnutrition in low- and middle-income countries drives the obesity pandemic. The World Health Organization (WHO) indicated that 1.9 billion adults were overweight (39%) worldwide, of whom more than 600 million (13%) were obese. An additional 42 million children under 5 years old were overweight or obese. Much of the disease burden today lies in Asia, where about half of overweight and obese children live. Yet even in Africa the number rose from 5.4 to 10.6 million children between 1990 and 2014.

How beauty is differently perceived around the world with regards to body weight, shape, and size is rooted in culture and tradition, race and ethnicity, social class and gender. And fat is (still) a feminist issue in many ways, the thesis of Susie Orbach's 1978 work, though this idea is beyond the scope of this book. Nevertheless, obesity carries with it an increased risk of many chronic diseases (e.g., type 2 diabetes mellitus [T2DM], heart disease), though the degree to which it impacts almost all body organs and systems is underappreciated. Hypertension, stroke, pulmonary diseases, non-alcoholic fatty liver diseases, depression, infertility, polycystic ovary syndrome, osteoarthritis, gout, and several cancers are all associated with obesity. And, in many places, discrimination and weight bias toward overweight and obese adults and children is common; children are often bullied, and adults frequently suffer a broad range of social and economic consequences.

Who suffers from chronic diseases, and what are the leading causes of death globally?

The average life span in the US rose to 79.1 years in 2014, up 5 years since 1980. Even so, approximately 1 in 2 adults has at least one chronic illness, of whom 25% have resulting limitations in daily activities and functioning. And more than 7 in 10 deaths annually are due to chronic diseases, of which heart disease, cancer, and stroke account for more than 50%. Yet there are great inequalities in disease burden, with the highest percentage of avoidable deaths from heart disease, stroke, and hypertension occurring among black men in the southern US. Health disparities are not innate but, rather, reflect differences in income that influence both access to healthcare and behaviors (like diet, physical activity, and smoking). As a result, gains in longevity are not evenly distributed in the US, a reflection of increasing disparities in income across race/ethnicity, socioeconomic status, and region. A 2017 study indicated that life expectancy among those born in the Mississippi Delta and on Native American reservations in either Dakota was around 70 years, for example; conversely, those on the California coast were expected to reach 85 years. Yet, chronic diseases are no longer restricted to high-income nations: the demographic and economic shifts that occur as regions move from agrarian to industrial then technologic societies bring an increase in noncommunicable diseases (NCDs), like heart disease, T2DM, stroke, and cancer. The leading cause of death *globally* was heart disease in 2016, compared to diarrheal diseases in 1990 (the latter due mainly to infectious disease and maternal and child malnutrition). The ongoing Global Burden of Disease Study showed substantial decreases in communicable diseases across all levels of socioeconomic status and an increase in the percentage of older adults worldwide, including those above age 90. WHO estimated that approximately 17.7 million people died from cardiovascular diseases (CVD) in 2015, including both heart disease and stroke, 31% of all global deaths. While NCDs remain more common in high- compared to low- and medium-income countries—88% versus 37%—more than 3 in 4 NCD deaths occur in low- and middle-income countries.

Despite the rapid increase of NCDs in low- and middle-income countries, 52% of deaths are still due to communicable (infectious) diseases, many a result of maternal and child malnutrition, compared to only 7% in high-income countries. India, comprising 18% of the global population (1.34 billion) and 2000 ethnic groups spread across 29 states and 7 union territories, is an exemplar. The prevalence of NCDs increased substantially from 1990 to 2016, with heart disease overtaking diarrheal diseases during this time frame. Yet tremendous variability occurs across the country, with lower-income states facing a continuing high prevalence of infectious disease, maternal and child mortality, and malnutrition-related deficiencies and diseases alongside increasing chronic diseases. The concurrence of conditions related to both undernutrition and overnutrition in India as well as China and the African continent is what WHO calls the "double burden of malnutrition." In these regions, diseases like vitamin A deficiency and stunting coexist within populations, and even within families, alongside diseases like obesity and heart disease. Together, these difficult public health challenges create extreme health burdens for those affected and astronomical healthcare costs for governments. Unlike most communicable diseases caused by a single infectious agent, NCDs result from a complex interplay of factors. While genetic predisposition matters, WHO estimates that a whopping 80% of all heart disease, stroke, and T2DM cases—and over 40% of cancers—can be prevented through lifestyle factors like diet. Moreover, WHO recently concluded that poor diet is *the leading risk factor* responsible for the global burden of disease and ill health.

What are the causes of food poisoning, and how can it be reduced?

Foodborne illnesses are caused by pathogenic microorganisms like bacteria, viruses, and parasites (as well as chemicals and toxins, both naturally occurring and synthetic). "Food poisoning" symptoms vary from unnoticeable to mild, severe to fatal, a function of both the dose of the contaminant and the health and development of the affected individual. Infants, children, pregnant women, the elderly, and those sick or immunocompromised are most vulnerable and more likely to suffer from serious symptoms. And approximately one-third of foodborne illnesses occur in children under 5, creating a cycle of malnutrition and diarrhea responsible for a large proportion of childhood disease and death.

Bacteria, notably *Salmonella, Campylobacter,* and *Escherichia coli,* cause the majority of foodborne illness, often leading to a host of gastrointestinal conditions like abdominal pain, vomiting, and diarrhea; *Listeria* and *Vibrio cholerae* are rarer but often more serious. Common sources of these bacteria are un- or undercooked animal foods (including raw shellfish and eggs), unpasteurized (raw) milk, and fruits and vegetables contaminated with animal feces. Each of these bacterial illnesses can be treated with antibiotics, though effectiveness is currently being compromised due to the increasing prevalence of antibiotic resistance in some places (Chapter 12).

Hepatitis A and norovirus are common viral causes of foodborne illness, often a result of unsafe food handling; norovirus, associated with cruise ship buffets, is the leading cause of outbreaks in the US. Parasites like *Giardia* and *Cryptosporidium* may be transmitted from consuming vegetables and fruits contaminated via soil or water. Prions are a type of protein that, when mutated, cause various neurodegenerative diseases that are untreatable and fatal. One such disease, bovine spongiform encephalopathy (BSE), was first observed in cattle in the UK in the 1980s and later dubbed "mad cow disease." A variant of Creutzfeldt-Jakob disease linked to the consumption of BSE cows and other animals was first seen in 1996; it is extremely rare, with only 231 cases in 12 countries documented between 1994 and 2016, of which 222 were in the UK and other European countries where BSE is most prevalent. Though not commonly associated with foodborne illness, contamination from various chemicals in the environment, both natural (like cyanide) and synthetic (like dioxin), can also cause acute and chronic illnesses (Chapter 13).

The first major WHO report measuring the global burden of disease due to foodborne illness from 2005 to 2015 found that diarrheal diseases were most common and mainly caused by *Norovirus, Campylobacter, E. coli,* or *Salmonella,* sickening an astounding 550 million people annually and causing 230 000 deaths. Those in Africa, Southeast Asia, and the eastern Mediterranean suffer the highest percentages of foodborne illness, as do those in lower-income regions. In the US, the Centers for Disease Control and Prevention (CDC) estimates that 48 million get sick, 128 000 are hospitalized, and 3000 die annually from foodborne illness.

While most cases strike groups of people within a community (e.g., a catered event, cafeteria meal, etc.), a small but growing percentage of cases occur across states, a function of food supply consolidation and improved detection, among other factors. Multistate outbreaks comprised 14% between 2001 and 2010 but caused a disproportionately high percentage of illnesses, hospitalizations, and deaths.

Raw (or undercooked) animal foods are most likely to be contaminated with foodborne pathogens in the US, including poultry, meat, shellfish, and eggs. Fresh produce, often consumed raw, is the leading cause of foodborne illness in absolute numbers; sprouts are a major culprit, a result of being grown in manure or cleaned with unsafe water. Unpasteurized beverages like fruit juices, cider, and milk (Chapter 4) also pose a risk. Organic farming methods do not eliminate the possibility of foodborne illness, and a small but increasing number of outbreaks have been traced to organic foods (due to increased production, not greater risk). Of 18 detected incidents in the US between 1992 and 2014, 4 were due to unpasteurized dairy products, 8 to produce, 2 to eggs, 2 to nut and seed products, and 2 to multi-ingredient foods.

Much foodborne illness is due to food consumed outside of the home, whether street fare in low- and middle-income nations or restaurant meals in more affluent countries. Proper hygiene and safe food handling among food workers are key as infected individuals can transmit a pathogen to unwitting eaters. CDC recommends four steps individual eaters can take to reduce the risk and spread of foodborne illness in the home: (1) **Wash hands** with warm, soapy water before and during food preparation, as well as surfaces, cutting boards, dishes, utensils, and the like; (2) **Separate raw foods** like meat, poultry, and seafood from others to prevent cross-contamination; (3) **Cook to kill** pathogens in animal foods by using a thermometer to measure internal temperature; and (4) **Chill food** within 2 hours to reduce or prevent bacterial growth, which is more likely to occur between 40 and 140°F.

A strong regulatory food safety framework both within and between nations is required to reduce foodborne illness alongside individual efforts. Collaboration between governments, nongovernmental organizations, food producers, and industry is required across the food supply chain. Though surveillance systems in the US have improved in recent years, better prevention efforts and more timely detection are needed. Because of the increasing globalization of the food supply in the past century, the Codex Alimentarius ("Food Code") Commission of FAO and the World Health Organization (WHO) was established in 1963 to provide standards, guidelines, and codes of practice surrounding a broad range of issues that include food hygiene and food safety (as well as food processing, additives, pesticides, antibiotics, labeling, and import/export issues surrounding trade).

How do agriculture and food production contribute to climate change?

The current climate change crisis is due to the high concentration of greenhouse gases (GHGs) that create a warming, or "greenhouse," effect when they are trapped in the lower atmosphere when radiating back from the Earth toward space. A panel of 1300 independent scientific experts from around the world concluded that there is a greater than 95% probability that rising temperatures across the globe are attributable to human ("anthropogenic") activities during the past 50 years, mainly due to GHGs. The panel further concluded that the three major GHGs responsible are carbon dioxide (CO_2, 76%), methane (CH_4, 16%), and nitrous oxide (N_2O, 6%). CO_2 results principally from the consumption of fossil fuel energy sources, which is particularly high in the food system (93%) compared to other sectors on average (86%).[2]

While fossil fuels burned for energy and heat production (25%) and transportation (14%) are the largest contributors of GHGs, agriculture also plays a big role. The US Environmental Protection Agency (EPA) estimated that 14% of GHG emissions (GHGe) in the US came from agriculture in 2007. Estimates rose to 24% in 2014 when combining agriculture, forestry, and other land uses, of which the cultivation of crops and livestock and deforestation (mainly for meat production) were the major contributors. Livestock-related GHGe contributed about two-thirds of all agricultural emissions between 2001 and 2010, which include enteric fermentation from methane-producing ruminant animals (40%), manure left on pasture (16%), and manure management (7%) (Chapter 12); remaining emissions came from synthetic fertilizers (13%), rice paddies (10%), and burning savannas (5%). Notably, agriculture can also help remove CO_2 from the atmosphere by sequestering carbon from soil, dead organic matter, and biomass.

Climate change is responsible for a host of environmental problems due to unpredictable weather patterns driven mainly by the dramatic average increase in temperatures across the globe. Temperature and precipitation fluctuations impact agricultural productivity, though studies show that effects vary due to myriad factors such as sensitivity to temperature, water, and CO_2, alongside expected variables like crop type, region, and production practices. A 2014 report from China, for example, found that temperature changes from 1980 through 2008 increased total yield for wheat (1.3%) and rice (0.4%) yet decreased maize by 12%. There is also growing evidence that the increased CO_2 in the atmosphere may be having a deleterious effect on the nutritional profile of crops. Higher CO_2 seems to lead to a higher carbohydrate composition in many plants but, in others, reduces concentrations of calcium, potassium, zinc, iron, and, for some crops, protein. Climate change can also impact the nutritional content of plants as a result of soil alterations that affect microbial activity and nutrient availability.[3]

While there may be ways to adapt global production to select for crops better suited to warmer temperatures, the unpredictability of weather patterns decreases farmers' ability to accurately plan for extreme weather events, which can wipe out entire harvests and compromise food security. Low- and middle-income regions are most vulnerable, especially those dependent on subsistence farming and with limited agricultural supports and safety nets, including those reliant on livestock in environments unsuitable for crops. A few reports even show an association between climate change and childhood stunting. There is much debate concerning to what degree climate change will influence agriculture: global yield may adapt and remain largely unchanged due to agronomic and technologic advances, while developments in plant physiology, genetics, and breeding may preserve nutritional content. Scientists are employing crop simulation models to better understand, and prepare for, potential impacts.

The international 2015 Paris Agreement, the first universal accord, was reached at the 21st session of the Conference of the Parties of the United Nations Framework Convention on Climate Change and adopted by 195 countries. (The US later withdrew, in 2017.) Its overarching goal was to address climate change globally in a way that keeps average temperatures "well below 2°C above pre-industrial levels." To this end, the member states aim to reduce CO_2 emissions by 50% by 2050 and 100% by 2100. Reducing reliance on fossil fuels across all sectors is critical—and possible. A 2007 report found that producing an "energy-deficient diet" that meets the minimum required calorie and nutrient targets of the Dietary Guidelines for Americans, for instance, decreased energy use within the food system by 74%.

Are fertilizers farming friend or foe?

Soil needs a number of key nutrients to produce crops, and fertilizers that provide nitrogen (N), phosphate (P_2O_5), and potassium (potash, K_2O) to enhance growth. A wide range of organic fertilizers including animal manure, guano (the accumulated excrement of seabirds and bats, particularly rich in these very nutrients), sewage sludge, and compost have been employed traditionally to maintain soil health and are still used in some food systems. "Cover crops" like peas, beans, lentils, and clover act as "green manure" to nourish soil and surrounding plants with their nutrients, which reduces the need for topical fertilizers; they also mitigate soil erosion by reducing runoff. But the discovery that led to the creation of N-based fertilizers in the early 20th century indelibly altered the course of agriculture, allowing direct application of inorganic N to the soil. About half of the world's fertilizer is N-based; Asia is by far the largest producer and consumer and Africa, the smallest. For sub-Saharan Africa in particular, it is cheaper to expand land to increase crop yield rather than apply costly fertilizers.

Fertilizer is indeed associated with improved productivity, coaxing higher crop yields for a given area of land. In the 1970s and 80s, for instance (following the Green Revolution, Chapter 3), fertilizers were believed responsible for producing half of India's cereal crop and one-third of cereals worldwide. N-based fertilizers are used predominantly for livestock feed and pastures, accounting for 50–70% of all use in major beef-producing countries including the US, UK, Canada, France, and Germany. (Corn-fed beef is particularly problematic due to its high N needs.) World demand for fertilizer is expected to grow about 1.6% annually through 2019, when it is expected to reach 199 million tons; N-based products will see the largest demand and growth.

The N cycle is a natural process essential to life—air is 78% N, for example—circulating between land- and water-dwelling animals and microorganisms and the atmosphere. There are thus many different chemical forms of N that play a role at various stages in agriculture. Notably, bacteria break down N in the soil into nitrates, which build up and sink into water tables, eventually reaching drinking water, streams, and oceans where they can impact both human and environmental health. (Phosphorus shares the same fate.) Buildup in soil also disrupts beneficial bacteria that can lead to an imbalance in minerals and organic matter that degrades soil quality over time, and soils replete in inorganic matter are particularly susceptible to erosion. Eroded soil holds fewer nutrients and less water, for example, both increasing water needs (hence irrigation that increases cost and stresses water tables) and reducing overall productivity over time. (Soil erosion is a result of many intensive farming practices related to monoculture, or growth of single crops, and other practices that reduce fertility, not just fertilizer use.) Excess atmospheric N that produces ammonia and ozone also contributes to air pollution that can create, or exacerbate, breathing problems, decrease visibility, and compromise plant growth.

Critically important is N_2O (nitrous oxide), a major GHG with about 310 times the global warming power of CO_2; it plays a major role in climate change. Agriculture is the single largest source of N_2O in the US, accounting for 75% of emissions in 2015, largely due to fertilizer use; breakdown of manure and urine from livestock contributes an additional 5%.

In aggregate, the excessive use of N-based fertilizers in farming has led to accumulations in land and water that have grave implications for sustainability. EPA calls this "nutrient pollution" and states it is "one of America's most widespread, costly, and challenging environmental problems." It is also a global problem—and growing.

What's the problem with pesticides?

Pesticides have largely supplanted manual tasks like weeding and setting animal traps to protect crops in major agri-food systems, which both reduce human labor and increase crop yield. These "crop protection chemicals" refer to any compound used to prevent, destroy, repel, or control an unwanted animal or plant from compromising crops. They can also be used as a regulator, defoliant, or desiccant or to stabilize N to promote growth. The term "pesticide" is often used generically, though it refers to four major categories based on intended target: insecticides (insects), rodenticides (rodents), fungicides (fungi), and herbicides (weeds). Of these, herbicides is the single greatest class. (There are numerous other pesticides employed for specific uses, including in nonfarming activities.) Pesticides are used in both conventional and organic farming systems (Chapter 4), the only difference being that the latter are biologically derived rather than synthetic (nonbiologically derived); they are sometimes referred to, more precisely, as biopesticides.

Pesticide use increased globally at a rate of about 11% per year, from 0.2 million tons in the 1950s to more than 5 million tons by 2000. Between 2005 and 2012, pesticide use remained level in the US, UK, and India but rose precipitously in China and Brazil. China is the largest consumer of pesticides, by far. The global pesticide market, dominated by a few multinationals, is approximately $50 billion. Because pesticides are inherently toxic and often nonspecific (i.e., kill unintended targets), they can deleteriously affect humans as well as other plant and animal life. Pesticides are assessed for safety and classified according to toxicity by individual nations and international bodies like WHO and FAO. Highly hazardous pesticides (HHPs) comprise a category with known acute and/or chronic effects in humans, particularly in children and farmworkers. Exposures are mainly due to regular occupational contact—handling, application, mixing, spraying, storage, disposal, and the like—but also to accidental or intentional poisonings. Exposure can also result from environmental contamination through food or water containing pesticide residues.

Those most at risk of poisoning are farmworkers, a result of persistent and high exposure to a broad range of pesticides. Many studies have shown that farmers have a higher risk of neurological, liver, and respiratory diseases as well as T2DM, some cancers, CVD, and Parkinson's. Chronic exposure to HHPs is particularly dangerous, affecting almost all organs and systems, including the blood, skin, eyes, nervous system, kidneys, cardiovascular system, gastrointestinal tract, reproductive system, liver, and endocrine system. Evidence is inconclusive as to whether pesticide exposure impacts the immune system. Recalling that a great many children work on farms, particularly in the developing world, it has been found in the past that some HHPs clearly led to childhood cancer, though such chemicals are no longer in use.

Farmers in low- and middle-income countries face increased health risks compared to those in high-income countries, a result of such factors as less stringent pesticide regulations, lack of proper training and education, inadequate monitoring, and use of outdated and more dangerous chemicals. HHPs in particular pose a far greater threat in low- and middle-income countries as they tend to be older, off-patent, cheaper, and readily available; these same pesticides are no longer on the market in high-income countries. There are approximately 200 000 acute pesticide-related deaths yearly, which does not include chronic illnesses; 99% of these occur in developing nations.

Integrated pest management (IPM) agriculture grew out of the awareness of the deleterious effect of pesticide overuse on farmers in particular, as well as the growing environmental hazards of pesticide resistance. FAO and WHO define IPM as

> the careful consideration of all available pest control techniques and subsequent integration of appropriate measures that discourage the development of pest populations and keep pesticides and other interventions to levels that are economically justified and reduce or minimize risks to human and animal health and/or the environment. IPM emphasizes the growth of a healthy crop with the least possible disruption to agro-ecosystems and encourages natural pest control mechanisms.

IPM utilizes both natural and synthetic pesticides when warranted and is a central part of FAO's agricultural programs in the developing world. While IPM is a complex and time-intensive process that needs to be adapted to individual farming situations, studies have shown that it benefits human health, the environment, and farm profitability.

Pesticide residue can reach eaters through food or water. Safety assessments are conducted regularly to ensure that exposures do not surpass the "maximum residue limits" threshold. In the US, EPA monitors pesticides used in food production, which are "GRAS" (i.e., generally recognized as safe). While residues can be detected in both organic and conventional produce—and are often somewhat higher in conventional produce—they are still lower than the maximum thresholds and pose no short-term human health risk according to comprehensive studies in the US and elsewhere. (Analyzing long-term health impacts is largely infeasible.) Washing produce in water may reduce exposures, as does peeling, though some pesticides are taken in through roots and are unaffected by these practices. Children are more susceptible to potential health risks from pesticide exposure due to incomplete development.

Nevertheless, the American Academy of Pediatrics (AAP) and others continue to recommend a diet rich in produce, *whether conventional or organic*, because the health benefits of consuming vegetables and fruits outweigh potential risk of pesticide exposure.

There are nonetheless differences of opinion on the health risks of pesticide residues. The Environmental Working Group (EWG), for example, expresses concern at even very low levels of exposure, especially for children and pregnant women. The group ranks produce according to those with the highest and lowest residues, suggesting buying organic when possible. Nonetheless, EWG concurs with AAP that eating more vegetables and fruits is the most important goal for individual health, however grown.

Glyphosate, an ingredient in Monsanto's Roundup—and the most widely used herbicide in the world—has received considerable research attention due to its pervasive use in agriculture on both traditional and genetically engineered (GE) crops. After decades of use, WHO ranked glyphosate as "probably carcinogenic in humans" in 2015 based on studies that showed tumors in animals, although supporting human data were limited: thus, the European Food Safety Authority (EFSA), WHO, and EPA agreed that glyphosate does not pose a risk at usual levels of exposure. In fact, FAO and WHO updated their conclusions on glyphosate in 2016, stating that glyphosate is "unlikely to pose a carcinogenic risk to humans from exposure in the diet."

Beyond the individual are the multifarious environmental effects of pesticides on soil, water, air, and biodiversity. Herbicides, for instance, initially decrease the number of weed species, impacting the ecological balance within natural habitats. Over time, however, excessive and/or chronic pesticide use can lead to resistance, leading to so-called superweeds that create new problems. Widespread aerosol application can also lead to drift. In 2017, an herbicide sprayed "over the top" (i.e., on growing plants rather than seeds) of GE herbicide-resistant crops spread to nearby fields of traditional (non-GE) produce, damaging 3.6 million acres of soybeans. Crops in 25 states using the herbicide were affected, with damage not only to soybeans but also cantaloupe, grapes, tomatoes, watermelon, and pumpkin—as well as home gardens, trees, and shrubs. Many herbicides have been associated with superweeds, whether applied to GE or traditional crops. But superweeds are a function of herbicide overuse and long predate the use of genetic engineering.

Pesticides vary in how rapidly they are degraded by soil, in many cases leading to long-term buildup that compromises soil health by decreasing the nutrients necessary for production. Pesticides are increasingly recognized as particularly damaging to the Earth, compromising soil structure and degrading soil fertility over time, in turn threatening future yields. Pesticides are also particularly problematic for oceans and waterways.

There are also numerous examples where pesticide residues, or those dispersed in air following mass spraying, have killed large numbers of bees, birds, small mammals, and amphibians. Insecticides like neonicotinoids, chemicals that damage the nervous system of consumers, have been related to colony collapse disorder of bees: there's been an approximate 50% reduction in honeybee populations since the early 1990s in both the US and the UK. Wild bees and managed bees are the single largest pollinator of crops; thus, their dwindling numbers pose a long-term threat to food security, though there have been some signs of recovery. (Neonicotinoids were banned in the European Union [EU] in 2013 but remain allowed in the US.)

There is little doubt that pesticides have protected crops worldwide, enabling the feeding of a growing population during the Green Revolution (Chapter 3). Their continued use is not sustainable, however: much research, including a UN 2017 special report, concludes that pesticides are not necessary to ensure future food security. The wide-ranging effects and negative externalities of pesticides in both the short and long term have led to increasing efforts to find alternatives like organic agriculture (Chapter 4), designed to protect the environment and people alike.

What is agriculture's role in water pollution and dead zones?

Agriculture uses about 92% of the freshwater on the planet, and about one-third relates to animal foods. The extensive use of pesticides in agriculture, which has increased 10-fold since the 1960s, impacts waterways through irrigation runoff, particularly in North America, Europe, and parts of South and East Asia. Nitrate is the most common pollutant in agriculture wastewater due to N-based fertilizer. Dangerous pesticides can also end up in water supplies in the developing world, where regulations aren't as strong. Studies have shown that manure waste often leaches into groundwater, leaving detectable traces of antibiotics, vaccines, and hormones that end up in drinking water.

A 2017 report on the impact of agricultural pollution on global water supplies estimates that 38% of water bodies are "significantly under pressure." Agriculture is responsible for substantial surface-water and groundwater pollution in China, and it is the main source of pollution in rivers and streams in the US. The accumulation of pollutants and nutrients (like salts, N, and phosphorus) in waterways damages soil en route, leading to erosion and salinization. Water also becomes over-enriched in nutrients (i.e., eutrophication), which spurs algal blooms that reduce oxygen, suffocate aquatic plants and animals, decrease biodiversity, disrupt ecosystems, and create "dead zones." FAO reports that 415 coastal areas globally are impacted by eutrophication, of which 169 were hypoxic in 2007 compared to 10 in 1960. One of the first dead zones identified was the Chesapeake Bay in the US in the 1970s, a result of factory and agricultural pollution; it is smaller today due to improved regulations, though still present. In August 2017, the US National Oceanic and Atmospheric Administration reported that the dead zone off the Gulf of Mexico, near the delta of the Mississippi River, is about the same size as the state of New Jersey (8776 square miles), its largest since 1985. The majority of the world's dead zones are on US coasts, in the Baltic Sea, and off of Japan and the Korean Peninsula.

What is the state of seafood, and why does overfishing matter?

Fishing tools and technology have become even bigger and more powerful in the past century. Single fishing lines have been replaced by so-called longlines containing many thousands of hooks, individual traps became a system of hundreds, and enormous lattices replaced small nets. As a result, today's commercial fishers are capable of catching ever-increasing numbers of fish at one time. This, in combination with historically lax regulations on quotas, has led to overfishing, in which more fish are caught than can be replaced through natural reproduction. Overfishing depletes the ocean's resources and, in so doing, compromises livelihoods, threatens biodiversity, and decreases food security. Numerous species have faced extinction throughout human history, including the Atlantic cod and the giant bluefin tuna. Bluefin tuna fishing, for example, now uses advanced GPS systems that spot the fish from afar for easy capture; they are caught in gigantic nets and shot, hardly what one thinks of as "fishing".[4]

Overfishing of any species leads to another major problem: by-catch. By-catch refers to the incidental capture of unwanted species (e.g., fish, turtles, corals, marine mammals, sponges, seabirds), which die during capture or on board and are then discarded. The shrimp industry is particularly egregious, with some estimates suggesting that for every 1 pound of shrimp caught up to 6 pounds of other species are discarded. Though difficult to measure, some estimates suggest that as much as 40% of the world's catch is by-catch, or 63 billion pounds. In the US, by-catch estimates in 2014 were 17–22%, a result of increased efforts to address the problem.

The World Wildlife Fund (WWF) currently estimates that more than 85% of the world's fisheries have been pushed to the point of collapse or have already collapsed. It summarizes myriad reasons why restoring and sustaining oceans and waterways is so critical, providing social and economic benefits among those in coastal communities for whom fishing is a livelihood; nutrition and health benefits to eaters as seafood is a major contributor to essential protein intake for billions; and environmental benefits to ocean ecosystems, vital for maintaining natural systems that ensure that sea life may thrive and reproduce, which ensures food security. Global changes in fishing regulations and practices are underway to restore fishery stocks and wildlife populations; aquaculture (Chapter 13) may be part of the solution. But poor fishery management, illegal fishing, paucity of wildlife and marine system protections, subsidies, and inadequate support for fishers and communities where livelihoods are compromised remain challenging issues to create the changes in the commercial fishing industry necessary to replenish and sustain wild populations.

Curbing and controlling overfishing and pollution are critical aspects of the Paris Agreement to combat climate change. Still, Fen

Montaigne of *National Geographic* implores that "the fundamental reform that must precede all others is not a change in regulations but a change in people's minds. . . . Only when fish are seen as wild things deserving of protection, only when the Mediterranean bluefin is thought to be as magnificent as the Alaskan grizzly or the African leopard, will depletion of the world's oceans come to an end." Expanding our global palate to include a broader array of seafood beyond a few species is paramount, as is turning to those at the lower end of the food chain that contribute to restoration of waterways, like oysters and others. Decreasing reliance on animal proteins, including seafood, and increasing plant protein consumption will also help.

What are the causes and impacts of food waste?

It is difficult to conceive that 30–50% of edible food is wasted worldwide, approximately 1.3 billion tons annually worth about $1 trillion. Proportion varies by food group and region, though FAO estimates that a staggering 45% of all fruit and vegetables, 35% of seafood and fish, 30% of cereals, 20% of dairy products, and 20% of meat go uneaten.

FAO defines "food waste" as any nutritious and safe food diverted from human consumption. Both plant and animal foods are wasted at every step of their life cycle, beginning with damage during production, harvesting, postharvest handling, and storage; edible food is also sometimes left to rot on fields if selling isn't economically worthwhile. Food processing activities of all kinds create food waste, often when only some parts of the whole food are utilized, like juicing citrus fruit. Whether ending up at local markets, wholesalers, supermarkets, or big box stores, much food is lost during postharvest storage and transportation, particularly in developing nations where technologies are inadequate for moving food safely from farm to market to consumer, a result of an insufficient "cold chain." Food waste also occurs at the retail level, where food may be discarded due to inadequate customer demand, the "ugly fruit" syndrome. Further loss can also happen from transporting food from retail to household and, finally, during household consumption.

Food waste occurs everywhere. In developing nations, about 40% is lost during production, harvesting, processing, and transport. In middle- and high-income countries, a comparable proportion is lost at the consumption level. Indeed, 42% of food waste occurs at the household level in the EU, similar to the figure for the US. Data aggregated from the US, Canada, Australia, and New Zealand found that the foods most wasted by consumers were seafood (33%), fruits and vegetables (28%), grain products (27%), milk (17%), and meat (12%). Americans toss almost 300 pounds of food per person annually, costing about $1500 for a family of 4 and adding up to as much as $218 billion as a country. A study of urban food waste in New York, Denver, and Nashville found that 3.5 pounds of food were wasted per person weekly, two-thirds of it edible; around 10% wasted food because they didn't want to eat leftovers (!).

Other studies suggest that confusion about "sell by" and "best by" dates—misunderstood (and confusing) manufacturing terms unrelated to safety—also plays a role, leading consumers to discard food that is harmless and nutritious. Despite the growing media attention about the magnitude of food waste, 76% believe they waste less food than the average American, suggesting room for knowledge and behavior change. Remarkably, the same study found that diverting discarded food into hungry mouths—known as "food rescue"—could create 68 million meals, enough to feed 46% more people in Denver, 48% in Nashville, and 26% in New York. Diverting food waste by reducing loss along food production chains (notably, through improving cold chains in the developing world and developing infrastructure) and reducing consumer and retail waste in high-income nations will also curtail dramatically the need to increase yields in future decades.

Food waste carries with it other solemn impacts beyond the moral issue of discarding nourishment in a world where so many are hungry. FAO estimates that 28% (1.4 billion hectares) of the land used for agriculture annually is spent to grow food that is wasted, and the water cost of wasted food is 250 km^3, or 3 times the volume of Lake Geneva. Discarded food creates a significant portion of municipal solid waste in landfills, where it generates methane, a greenhouse gas yielding 3.3 billion tons of CO_2 equivalents contributing to climate change; meat waste is particularly damaging. Fuel, animal feed, fertilizer, pesticides, labor, and other unrecovered costs are also embedded in the price of food waste. Because of the higher inputs of producing meat and animal products compared to plant foods (Chapter 12), tossing such foods is particularly wasteful of finite natural resources.

Part II

DINING THROUGHOUT HUMAN HISTORY

SCIENCE, TECHNOLOGY, EATER, ENVIRONMENT

Species of all kinds, including our own, forge relationships with the natural environment to nourish themselves. Over the course of millions of years, human beings have made scientific discoveries and developed tools and technologies enabling novel ways of producing and consuming food. Contemporary eaters navigate the built environment for food—supermarkets, food courts, cafeterias, restaurants, and the like—rather than the farm, and savvy eaters need to sift science from junk science to make healthy and sustainable choices.

3

HOW REVOLUTIONS, DISCOVERIES, AND INVENTIONS SHAPE OUR DIET

PALEO TO PRESENT

What is the Paleolithic diet? What did hunter–gatherers actually eat?

While "Paleo" diets may seem to be a 21st-century fad, the concept has solid scientific roots in the disciplines of evolutionary biology and anthropology. The first article discussing the diet of early humans from a nutritional perspective appeared in the *New England Journal of Medicine* in 1985, and many studies since then have examined the potential merits of the Paleolithic diet for people in our own time.

Indeed, more than 99% of our history has been spent as hunter–gatherers, beginning with the emergence of bipedal primates (hominins) with *Australopithecus afarensis* 3.85–2.95 million years ago. The "Stone Age" period of the Paleolithic era began around 2.4 million years ago with "handy man" *Homo habilis*. Paleoanthropologists estimate that *Homo sapiens*—anatomically modern humans, our own species—emerged in Africa during the Middle Paleolithic, approximately 200 000–300 000 years ago. Fossil records indicate that the diet of bipedal primates, and, much later, *H. sapiens*, included leaves, seeds, roots, nuts, fruit, and water. Insects may have contributed, alongside small invertebrates (e.g., lizards). Wild grains would have played a very minimal role as they are small, hard, and difficult to digest when raw. Later, hominins may have consumed wild eggs. Honey was discovered during this time, too, though it was available only in certain regions and at certain times. Early hunter–gatherers probably stumbled across wine a result of overripened and fermented fruit, though consumption would have been extremely limited and by (happy) chance; newer scientific evidence suggests that monkeys discovered the pleasurable effects of alcohol in exactly the same way.

There is thus much evidence to suggest that the foundation of hunter–gatherer diets was in fact plants, not animals, which is also akin to the diets of chimpanzees and apes, our closest primate relatives.[1] Perhaps "gatherer–hunterer" is more accurate: while today's "Paleo diet" involves piling on meat, our ancestors were likely the consumers of a plant-based diet. Moreover, scavenging played a larger role than hunting in early diets. The role of land- and water-dwelling animals shot up to around 1.5 million years ago as hunting capabilities improved due to increasingly sophisticated and varied stone tools such as bows and arrows and spear-throwers.

Building fires was likely a significant factor in our evolving diet: cooking predigests raw food, in a sense, making it easier to consume and absorb nutrients. Some scientists hypothesize that cooking freed up energy from the gastrointestinal tract, thereby enabling calories for other activities and fueling larger brain growth. Indeed, anthropological records suggest that the evolution of the bigger-brained species *Homo erectus* about 2 million years ago coincides with the control of fire.[2]

Interestingly, recently unearthed stone tools across settlement spots in Europe from more than 30 000 years ago show residues of heated wild grains including oat, cattail, and fern. The tool perhaps would have been used to crush grain in a bowl, a prehistoric mortar and pestle. Whether it was mixed with water to create porridge is anyone's guess, but it is clear that grains were used to some degree during the Mid-Upper Paleolithic as early humans gained experience and skill working with tools and fire to further dietary diversity.

While hominins populated the planet, diets took on an increasingly local flair, utterly dependent on what geography, climate, and season offered. (And sheer luck.) People gradually learned what was safe for consumption and what wasn't, which tastes provided pleasure and which did not, providing ever greater variability in our increasingly omnivorous diet. Hence, there was no single "Paleo" diet: the proportion of plants and animals consumed varied across groups, just as they do in modern hunter–gatherer diets, a dietary flexibility required for survival. But what is clear is that the Paleolithic diet of yore bears little resemblance to contemporary diets of *H. sapiens*, filled with sugar, salt, fat, and high-calorie, highly processed foods. For these reasons, some scientists have put forth the "evolutionary discordance" hypothesis, which posits that diets today are out of sync with how our genome evolved and should better resemble hunter–gatherer diets for optimal health, weight, and disease prevention; these beliefs have brought the Paleo diet back in style once again (Chapter 4).

What is the Neolithic Revolution, and how did diets change after the birth of agriculture?

The Neolithic period, or "New Stone Age," began around 10 000 BCE. Somewhere around this time, a group of *H. sapiens* arrived in what is now known as the Fertile Crescent, located in the modern-day Middle East. Anthropological remains indicate this is where early humans began cultivating wild wheat. An earlier and similar settlement has also been identified in southwestern Asia, where barley and millet were cultivated. During this time, *H. sapiens* began interacting with nature in ways not previously seen, learning to manage air, water, and temperature to cultivate food in a time also described as the (first) agricultural revolution.

Over time, tools and technologies enabled more efficient growing, reaping, harvesting, and storing of grains. Humans eventually mastered plants like beans, nuts, vegetables, and fruit, and began selecting them for desired traits. The Neolithic era also marks the beginning of animal husbandry (notably, cows, sheep, goats, and chickens); humans may have begun raising animals specifically for their milk 5000–6000 years ago. Around the same time, *H. sapiens* learned that some plant foods yielded oils that could be used for consumption (as well as lubrication and other uses).

Wine and beer also entered the diet during the Neolithic era. The initial discovery of beer was likely by chance, as with wine. Humans didn't learn to brew beer until about 4000 BCE, though winemaking likely began about 7400 years ago; mead-making, from honey, would have occurred somewhere in there as well. It wasn't until about 800–1300 CE that humans in the Near East, China, and Europe began distilling alcohol. Other additions to the diet included salt in China around 6000 BCE; sugar was first used as a sweetener in India around 500 BCE.

While the burgeoning food supply fueled the population explosion during this time—from 2–4 million to around 25 million—anthropological evidence suggests that humans were overly reliant on grains, resulting in a lack of nutritional diversity that compromised health. They were also at risk of food shortages when nature did not comply. As a result, the scientific consensus is that Neolithic humans had poorer health and shorter life spans than hunter–gatherers—bigger brains notwithstanding. They also had a greater risk of infectious disease, likely a result of the closer proximity to fellow humans and animals in growing settlements.

These observations led some experts to further examine the effects of the rise of agriculture, with one writer's trenchant quip, "Was it even a good idea?" In fact, the Neolithic "revolution" actually occurred over many thousands of years, in some cases *after* hunter–gatherers had settled into bountiful areas replete with wild plants, fish, and land animals.[3] Agriculture was also labor-intensive, leading to the use of slaves and creating social divisions that were increasingly complex, gendered, and stratified. All were major departures from hunter–gatherer lifestyles, which in many cases value egalitarianism and the sharing of food and social responsibilities. For these reasons and others, a number of historians single out the first agricultural revolution as one of the worst mistakes in human history (!).

It is unknown what in particular led humans to ultimately choose agriculture over hunter–gatherer lifestyles. Neolithic settlements rose and collapsed over thousands of years, often existing in concert with hunter–gatherer lifestyles and foraging civilizations. Yet agriculture in time won out—and still dominates food procurement.

How and why did the Industrial Revolution
impact food production?

The Industrial Revolution (IR) spanned the mid-18th to late 19th centuries. Countries began investing heavily in agriculture (e.g., the US Department of Agriculture [USDA] was founded in 1862). Synthetic gradually replaced natural fertilizers, and new methods were created to feed people beyond the farm. We learned how to harness power first from water, and then from steam. Inventions like tractors and plows made it easier to farm larger areas with less human labor. Similar changes came to the fishing industry: human- and wind-powered boats were eventually replaced with those running on steam and, later, the internal combustion engine. And, as in farming, fishing tools became bigger and more powerful. Steamships and, later, trains transported food from farms to cities.

While preserving fish or meat with salt had been practiced for millennia, it wasn't until the IR that large-scale food processing (Chapter 4) began to create shelf-stable food safe for future consumption. One notable example is canning,[4] which began in 1795; by 1870, canned foods were being produced en masse to feed soldiers and city dwellers. Still, the massive increase in urban populations made getting food safely to people challenging: demand exceeded supply, and in-home refrigeration did not yet exist. Foods were sometimes filled with toxic fillers—food adulteration—including lead in tea and "swill milk".[5] Public health legislation began to regulate the nascent food industry, and the sale of contaminated milk (for instance) was prohibited in 1861; cow's milk also became safer following pasteurization. (Interestingly, much of the public opposed pasteurization, a harbinger of the resistance shown still today to new food technologies.)

Another example demonstrating the tensions between the growing food system and public health in the US was the meatpacking industry c. 1850. Warehouses were unsafe and unsanitary, leading to the 1906 Pure Food and Drug Act and the Meat Inspection Act. Food- and waterborne illnesses were also common, and particularly impacted pregnant women and children. Even so, humans began living longer throughout the 19th and early 20th centuries, in part due to the control of infectious diseases.

During this period, the food industry continued finding new ways to accommodate changing lifestyles. Food was less likely to come directly from a farm than from a neighborhood supermarket filled with processed foods that decreased the effort of making meals from scratch. In 1916, the first supermarket, Piggly Wiggly, opened in Memphis, Tennessee, enabling customers to make independent selections. And the first fast food restaurants, A&W in 1919 and White Castle in 1921, further enabled the populace to procure ready-to-eat food outside of the home, a trend that continues today.

What is the Green Revolution, and how did it impact human health and the environment?

The early decades of the 20th century saw two world wars and the Great Depression, leading to widespread food shortages and hunger. Significant advances in agriculture followed, culminating in the "Green Revolution" (GR), a phrase coined in 1968. Crop breeding to improve yields was at the heart of the GR, initially with Dr. Norman Borlaug's semi-dwarf wheat (1944) that was more resistant to disease, and then with rice.[6] Corn and soybean yields also increased, in part for the growing meat and dairy industries that had been slowly turning to grain rather than grass for feed. Techniques for refining oils and sugars from these grains—like soybean oil and high-fructose corn syrup—began to play a prominent role in the Western food supply. The use of synthetic fertilizers and mechanized irrigation systems also exploded to optimize efficiency.

Another notable change was the increased size of farms, many of which became dedicated to one particular crop (i.e., "monoculture"). As well, growing efforts were devoted to seed, fertilizer, food processing, transportation, retail, and waste management. The portmanteau "agribusiness" was thus coined in 1957 to reflect the idea that traditional agriculture was part of a much larger food system with myriad players responsible for food, from farm to fork.

Despite productivity and food supply gains, many GR practices were later found to be hazardous to animal and human health, stimulating public health action and stronger regulations in the chemical industry. DDT, a synthetic insecticide introduced in the 1940s, is an intriguing example,[7] though there were numerous other infractions leading to calls for less damaging, more sustainable agricultural practices that still resound today.

What is the Genetic Revolution, and how did it affect food production?

The act of selecting crops for desired traits has doubtless been around since the earliest days of agriculture, though—as in so many cases throughout history—the reasons for the effects (the mechanism, in science-speak) were unknown. James Watson and Francis Crick's 1953 discovery of deoxyribonucleic acid (DNA), which encodes our genetic makeup, revolutionized scientific disciplines across the board. Food producers soon jumped on the bandwagon, and, in 1994, the first genetically engineered (GE) food came to market, a tomato bred to prolong shelf life and flavor through the addition of a second tomato gene that slowed rotting. Despite this early effort to create a GE food that benefits consumers, so-called first-generation crops designed primarily for farmers and food producers dominated the following decades. In 1996, the first GE seeds designed to be herbicide-tolerant or insecticide-resistant (or both) were planted. GE seeds were planted on 4.7 million acres in 1995, rising to 4.85 billion acres in 2015. They are now used in 28 countries worldwide, and the US, Brazil, Argentina, India, and Canada are the leading producers. In 2016, the vast majority of US soybeans (94%) as well as corn and cotton (around 75% each) were made using biotechnology. On average, seeds have reduced pesticide and herbicide application use. Some GE herbicide-tolerant crops have led to the development of superweeds, which become resistant to the chemical initially used to kill it and hence more robust—though this phenomenon can occur whenever herbicide is used, including among non-GE crops.

A great many foods in contemporary diets—depending on the country where you live and its legislation regarding biotechnology—are made with soybean oil, corn syrup, and the like. As a result, humans have been eating foods made with GE ingredients since the late 1990s. At the same time, the second-generation GE crops, which are created with the consumer in mind, have been slow to reach the market due to public discomfort with biotechnology. Yet despite the heated politics and rampant junk science surrounding GE, the major health and science organizations in the US and around the world—including the World Health Organization (WHO), the Food and Agriculture Organization of the United States (FAO), the European Food Safety Authority (EFSA), Center for Science in the Public Interest, and the Natural Resources Defense Council—have all independently concluded that foods resulting from genetic engineering are no less safe than those grown using traditional breeding methods. While each new crop requires individual safety assessment, the method itself does not appear inherently harmful. A newer technique called CRISPR (i.e., clustered regularly interspaced short palindromic repeats, pronounced "crisper") "snips" DNA at specific locations to remove undesirable traits, which enables faster, easier, and more precise modification without adding foreign genes. (See also Chapters 4 and 18.)

How have the Digital Revolution and Information Age impacted our diet?

Computing developments were underway in government and the military during the 1950s and 60s, and computers were increasingly used in businesses in the 1980s. Digital technology began supplanting mechanical and analog technology in electronics, the hallmark of the digital revolution (DR), sometimes referred to as the Third Industrial Revolution. The DR is considered one of the greatest achievements of humankind, comparable in magnitude to traveling to the moon. It has evoked widespread changes throughout society, including in food production and farming (Chapter 18).

The Information Age also altered how consumers procure food. The majority of Americans still shop in a traditional store: a 2017 Gallup poll reported that 83% go to supermarkets weekly, compared to only 4% who buy groceries online. But a growing proportion of individuals, particularly Millennials and Generation Z, relies upon the Internet to feed themselves. "Click and pick up" is increasingly popular, rather than traversing supermarket aisles on foot. Online shopping is expected to grow substantially in coming years; Amazon started delivering Whole Foods groceries in select cities in early 2018, for example—in under 2 hours.

Online food shopping is even bigger elsewhere. Nielsen's 2015 survey of 30 000 Internet users in 60 countries found that 25% of respondents currently buy groceries online; the highest proportions of users are in the Asia-Pacific region (China in particular), Africa/Middle East, and Latin America, and the lowest are in Europe and North America. Tesco launched the first virtual supermarket in South Korea in 2011, and others have followed. According to consumer behavior guru Nielsen, it is the era of "connected commerce" in which the virtual and physical worlds are blended to meet individual needs for personalization and convenience.

Dining out looks different today, too. Computers increasingly allow customers to make choices without human interaction in quick-service dining, and menus at sit-in spaces may be electronic rather than hard copy. And many search the Internet for a restaurant that best fits their needs, whether the latest hot spot or a place accommodating unique food preferences (like farm to table, or vegan).

At the same time, people today are increasingly interested in the role of food in health and sustainability, many of whom rely upon the Internet. Social media and smart phone apps enable connecting with online communities dedicated to specific food issues. The sky's the limit, whether for a supportive weight loss group or an activist-oriented organization dedicated to ethical eating. Access to copious information doesn't always lead to better food choices, alas: junk science imbues the food and nutrition world, filling newsfeeds with misinformation that often confuses rather than clarifies.

The kitchen itself is slowly evolving to reflect the times too, just as it did in prior eras. Meals created using 3D food printers were first conceived by NASA in 2013 as a way to provide safe and tasty food to astronauts on long space journeys and became a reality in 2016, beginning with pizza. Printers in home kitchens are scarce but were first used in some sports arenas, theme parks, and the like in 2017. Digital technology continues to change the kitchen environment in other ways as well, allowing communication via the "Internet of Things" (Chapter 18).

What are the top food inventions and technologies that have shaped how we eat and drink throughout human history?

Our journey from the Paleolithic era to the present is an astounding story of how biological requirements for food and water to sustain life, combined with human curiosity, led to experiential and scientific discoveries of how best to meet these basic human needs. Several inventions have already been highlighted, and Table 3.1 includes additional developments that indelibly impact the relationship among humans, the environment, and health still today.

The top-rated invention, home refrigeration, is one many people today take for granted, though the large cooling units in our home are among the more recent developments. Refrigeration keeps food safe to eat for longer periods of time, easing the ability to feed families on fewer resources, with less time dedicated to daily food procurement. The technology was developed during the mid-19th century and modified for home use in 1913. It didn't really take off until

Table 3.1 Top 20 Inventions in the History of Food and Drink[a]

1. Refrigeration
2. Pasteurization/sterilization
3. Canning
4. Oven
5. Irrigation
6. Threshing machine/combine harvester
7. Baking
8. Selective breeding/strains
9. Grinding/milling
10. Plough
11. Fermentation
12. Fishing net
13. Crop rotation
14. Pot
15. Knife
16. Eating utensils
17. Cork
18. Barrel
19. Microwave oven
20. Frying

[a]From The Royal Society (the UK National Academy of Sciences), 2012.

the 1930s, a sign of social progress and the rise of the middle class following the Great Depression and World War I. Today, almost all American homes have at least one refrigerator—and about 25% own two. Refrigeration is still changing lives for the better, especially among women: ownership worldwide skyrocketed from 24% in 1994 to 88% in 2014, though only 45% have a unit in Peru and 27% in India. *The Economist* notes that "[f]ridges are transforming women's lives in India and other emerging markets, just as they did in developed countries decades ago."

Many "top" inventions found in most home kitchens are commonplace and include canned foods, an oven, and a microwave, not to mention cooking tools like pots and utensils that've been around for millions of years. Other technologies are quietly incorporated to make our foods safer. Pasteurization (Chapter 4), for instance, is viewed as one of the greatest public health achievements of the 20th century and has saved countless lives. Others are related to food production, technologies born during the Neolithic Revolution that are still feeding today's growing population. Selective breeding is currently number eight on this list, and one might wonder whether genetically modified organisms will be added in the future. Will genetic engineering, much like Borlaug's semi-dwarf wheat, one day be thought responsible for saving billions of lives, whether from starvation or chronic disease?

4

CONTEMPORARY FOOD PRODUCTION, BUZZWORDS, AND POP NUTRITION

FACT OR FICTION?

What are "processed" foods, and how do they fit into a healthy diet?

Food processing transforms raw agricultural crops into food products. For many, "processed foods" carries a pejorative connotation, bringing to mind an array of snacks designed to tempt consumers' taste buds, like potato chips: raw potatoes are washed, sliced, fried, and packaged with preservatives—each a form of food processing—to keep them fresh and safe (and delicious) for eating.

There are many different food processing methods, from familiar kitchen activities (e.g., chop, mix, cook, grind, bake, freeze, can, pickle) to specific laboratory techniques (e.g., ferment, pasteurize, irradiate, homogenize, dehydrate), all of which alter food in some way or another. And there are additional reasons food is processed beyond simply making appetizing and convenient food people enjoy, often through the addition of flavors and other ingredients like salt, fat, and sugar. According to the Food Marketing Institute, an average American supermarket included 39 500 items in 2015, up from 8948 in 1975. More than 20 000 new products appeared in retail in 2016, and a vast majority of these were ultra-processed foods and beverages. Still, much food processing is done simply to keep foods safe, prolong shelf life, preserve or enhance nutrient content (nutrification, Chapter 6), and prevent foodborne illness. In fact, very few foods are *not* processed in some way in today's 21st-century global food supply. These include a plethora of pantry staples like ready-to-eat cereal, peanut butter, bread, canned tomatoes, and coffee that make eating easy and convenient (and often more pleasant). Even fresh fruit in the supermarket has undergone some processing, including washing, sorting, and perhaps a light (edible, tasteless) wax to prolong shelf life. A 2012 study conducted by four science-based organizations (Academy of Nutrition and Dietetics, American Society for Nutrition, Institute of Food Technologists, International Food Information Council) found little difference in healthfulness on average comparing nutrient intakes of 25 351 Americans across a broad range of processed food levels, likely due to the considerable variation within traditional categories. Other reports show that processed foods help people meet nutrition goals.

Studies like these demonstrate the ambiguity not in the research but, rather, the definition: processed food categories vary by country and organization (and researcher). In response, scientists reviewed various classification schemes and concluded that four categories— unprocessed/minimally processed, processed culinary ingredients, processed, ultra-processed—were most useful (Table 4.1).

The system underscores the importance of thinking about processed foods not as a binary (processed/unprocessed) but as a continuum. It also suggests, based on both the definitions and examples, that minimally processed foods are generally the most healthful. Yet studies in Australia, Brazil, Canada, New Zealand, Norway, Sweden, and the United States (US) have shown that ultra-processed foods dominate the food supply. One investigation, for instance, showed that 57.9% of energy intake among Americans was from ultra-processed foods, contributing 89.7% of added sugars to the diet. They also play an increasing role in low- and middle-income countries, where they can impact food production and trade; disrupt local and regional food systems; and displace traditional, more nutritious foods from the diet. Moreover, ultra-processed food often contributes more to environmental damage compared to those minimally processed through extensive processing and packaging

Table 4.1 The Continuum of Processed Foods

Processed Food Category	Definition and Example Methods	Example Foods	Nutrition Notes
Unprocessed/minimally processed foods	Plant or animal foods consumed shortly after harvest, slaughter, etc.; methods include wash, grate, peel, fillet, dry, debone, pasteurize, ferment (other than alcohol), dehydrate, freeze, can; products may have minimal packaging (e.g., bag, plastic wrap)	Fruit and vegetables that are fresh or preserved with nothing added, including bagged salads; fresh, frozen, or dried beans, legumes, and cereal grains; fresh squeezed or pasteurized 100% fruit or vegetable juice or dairy; raw and unsalted nuts and seeds; recognizable animal foods like meat, poultry, and fish; eggs; tea, coffee, and unsweetened water	Commonly referred to as "whole" foods (even if cut, peeled, frozen, pasteurized, etc. or milled simply to access the grain)
Processed culinary ingredients	Products in original form without added ingredients excepting additives to ensure shelf stability; methods include pressed, milled, ground, and purified	Sugars (e.g., white, maple syrup), animal fats and plant oils (like butter and canola oil), corn starch, flour, and salt	Cooking and baking staples that may be fortified (like salt and flour)

Table 4.1 Continued

Processed Food Category	Definition and Example Methods	Example Foods	Nutrition Notes
Processed	Modified whole foods, often with additional processed ingredients; methods include cans, jars, dehydration, brines, pickles, smoke, and salt	Canned, jarred, dried, pickled, and frozen fruits and vegetables that include sugar or other ingredients; tinned or smoked fishes (like tuna); cheese; deli meats (not reconstituted) like turkey, ham, and bacon; nuts (not raw)	Often more convenient than fresh whole foods and consumed as part of a meal or snack
Ultra-processed	Foods with additives, preservatives, fillers, etc. to prolong shelf life; methods include hydrogenation, hydrolysis, and reshaping	Bread, breakfast cereal, sweet and salty snacks, and canned soups; ready-to-eat or quickly prepared frozen burgers, fries, pizza; packaged baked goods and desserts; meat substitutes (soy, seitan, etc.); sugar-sweetened beverages (e.g., sodas, teas, fruit and milk drinks); and sweetened dairy products	Convenient foods usually consumed as is, often unrecognizable from whole foods; tend to be high in sugar, salt, refined grains, calories, and unhealthy fats and low in fiber and nutrients; fortified foods like diet meals and shakes and energy bars

that pollutes land, air, and water. One research group goes so far as to deem ultra-processed products a "world crisis."

The point may be hyperbolic but is not without some merit: the vast majority of ultra-processed foods are indeed less healthy overall, and sugar-packed beverages and breakfast cereals are exemplars. And ultra-processed foods contributed 21.2% of added sugars to the American diet, almost nine times more than processed foods (2.4%).

Nonetheless, there are instances within each processed food category that are more and less nutritious and/or have varying degrees of environmental impact—and many of us (myself included) enjoy ultra-processed foods whether due to taste, convenience, cost, or some other reason. Including more whole foods in the diet is sound advice, but getting science-savvy about nutrition (Parts III and IV) is the real key to creating a salubrious lifelong diet—not vilification and total denial.

Do red and processed meats cause cancer?

While definitions vary, the World Health Organization (WHO) defines red meat as "all mammalian muscle meat, including beef, veal, pork, lamb, mutton, horse, and goat." (No, pork is not "the other white meat," as US producers tout.) Processed meats begin with the base animal, usually pork or beef, and utilize salting, smoking, fermentation, and curing to enhance flavor, improve preservation, or both. Common examples range from deli meats (e.g., ham, turkey, pastrami, bologna, salami) to fast-food favorites (e.g., chicken nuggets, hot dogs, pepperoni), breakfast foods (e.g., bacon, sausage, blood pudding) to meat snacks (e.g., jerky, biltong). Processed meat often hides in meat-based dishes and sauces, too. SPAM—"Sizzle Pork and Mmm"—is an international exemplar with its six main ingredients: "pork with ham," salt, water, potato starch, sugar, and sodium nitrite. It came to market in 1937 and became a favored lunch for soldiers during World War II in Hawaii; it still holds a special place in Hawaiian cuisine but was gradually embraced by other states and, eventually, the world. There are now 15 varieties of SPAM sold in 43 countries—and 12.8 cans are eaten per second.

While processed meats are generally higher in salt, sugar, and preservatives than unprocessed meats, both are sources of saturated fat and heme iron. Some processing methods involve nitrites, which are metabolized into N-nitroso compounds in the body—and the same compounds are produced in the gut following red meat consumption. Smoked meats can lead to the formation of polycyclic aromatic hydrocarbons (PAHs), as can cooking red meat at high temperatures, like grilling; the latter methods also produce heterocyclic amines (HCAs). N-nitroso compounds, PAHs, and HCAs have all been shown to be cancer-promoting agents in numerous laboratory and animal studies, spurring human studies examining red and processed meats (RPM). And heme iron, the kind found predominantly in meat,[1] has been found to enhance HCA production through its metabolism, which may lead to deoxyribonucleic acid (DNA) mutations in the colon.

In 2014, the International Agency for the Research of Cancer (IARC) convened 22 experts from 10 countries to review more than 800 observational studies on RPM and cancer. The group concluded that processed meat was a group 1 agent (like tobacco) and carcinogenic. Specifically, 50 g of processed meat consumed daily increases colorectal cancer risk by 18%. The evidence is not as strong for red meat, with the IARC concluding it is "probably carcinogenic" in humans: 100 g of red meat consumed daily increases colorectal cancer risk by 17%. The IARC report led WHO to underscore its 2002 recommendation that people limit their consumption of RPM due to an increased risk of colorectal cancer. Many country-specific guidelines also recommend limiting RPM, and the American Institute of Cancer Research recommends avoiding processed meat and limiting red meat to less than 18 ounces weekly. Current studies are considering how the timing of intake across the life span, cooking method, and genetics impact the connection between RPM and colorectal cancer, while other research is examining associations with cancers like those of the prostate, stomach, and breast.

Are canned and frozen foods inferior to fresh?

Fresh produce is delightful, although it is more costly than canned and frozen, takes longer to prepare when cooking, and often goes to waste on household counters or refrigerator shelves. In fact, frozen and canned foods are also considered "whole foods"— or minimally processed—as long as additional elements aren't introduced (Table 4.1). A major preservative used in canning is salt, and most people consume too much; selecting no- or low-salt options is best. Meanwhile, many canned fruits swim in sweet syrup, adding extra calories from sugar. It is easier to find minimally processed frozen vegetables, fruits, and beans, though they can still include excess salt, sugar, and sauces. There's no need for guesswork: simply read the ingredients, nutrition facts panel, and calorie counts.

Produce is usually processed at its peak, flash-frozen at the same location where picked; this means maximal nutrients and vitamins are retained and maintained in your freezer. Thus, they can have even more vitamins and minerals compared to fresh produce that has been transported over a long period of time (particularly if conditions were suboptimal) or sitting around the market or house prior to consumption. Canning can lead to nutrient losses when vitamins leach into the liquid, just as when vegetables are boiled at home. But the amount lost is not significantly different from fresh produce that is not consumed immediately, which begins losing nutrients once picked. (The vegetable is, after all, dying.) Yet some canned foods have even more nutrients than fresh as heating and cooking increase the bioavailability of some nutrients. For example, canned tomatoes—the most frequently consumed canned vegetable in the US—have a higher lycopene content than fresh, an antioxidant shown to reduce the risk of prostate cancer in many studies.

The environmental footprint of frozen and canned foods is an additional consideration. Resources like fossil fuels are needed to create packaging, which ends up in landfills if nonrecyclable. Moreover, while materials science works to ensure that packaging is safe, knowledge is not always complete. Lead was originally used in canning, for example (as it was in paint and other household items), until the US Food and Drug Administration (FDA) prohibited it in 1995. Attention has since shifted to bisphenol A (BPA), which is used around the world to make epoxy resins that line some canned foods, and polycarbonate, a plastic used in beverage bottles, plastic storage containers, and other products. BPA was approved for use in the US in the 1960s, but research has emerged showing BPA can leach into food and liquids, especially when heated (like a warmed baby bottle or a water bottle sitting in the car on a very hot day). Animal studies have shown that BPA is a metabolic and endocrine disrupter that leads to a variety of poor health outcomes at high exposures, although evidence in humans at the levels commonly consumed, which are far less than these, is weak.

WHO, European Food Safety Authority (EFSA), Health Canada, FDA, and others continue monitoring BPA research for human safety concerns. An October 2016 EFSA report concluded, "BPA might affect the immune system in animals, but the evidence is too limited to draw any conclusions for human health"; the same conclusions were drawn regarding neurobehavioral and reproductive effects. A 2014 FDA report based on more than 300 studies between 2009 and 2013 reached similar conclusions. Even so, both EFSA and FDA reduced the tolerable daily intake, though noting that BPA was well below this level. Importantly, FDA and others had already prohibited the use of BPA in baby bottles, sippy cups, and other packaging given that infants and children are more vulnerable to toxicity.

In summary, scientists actively study the bioavailability of specific nutrients across a wide range of foods, comparing fresh to frozen to canned—and there are far too many examples to consider that vary across individual foods and the specific technology and storage conditions. Processing technologies are always advancing to preserve nutrient content and, when science warrants, reviewed to ensure safety. But the bottom line is that most people don't eat nearly enough vegetables and fruits for optimal health and disease prevention, and minimally processed foods help meet nutritional requirements. Research also shows that frozen foods from big box stores feed people with less expense, a critical consideration given that so many struggle to get supper on the table. Additionally, the market for products that minimize environmental impact is growing, enabling eco-conscious consumers to make greener choices. And many companies voluntarily change technologies to respond to consumer concerns; BPA has received considerable media attention, for example, and "BPA-free" packages are now available in many stores.

Are "natural," "raw," and "clean eating" concepts science, or nonsense?

The word "natural" is not meaningful when it comes to diet. Cyanide is natural, for example.

But it will still kill you. That's because cyanide is not just a substance synthesized for nefarious purposes like biological warfare. It is also found naturally in foods like almonds, particularly bitter almonds, as well as the pits of fruits like apricots and peaches. The amounts are generally too low to be concerning, demonstrating an indispensable scientific principle: the poison is in the dose. There are countless examples of this phenomenon, including in nutrition; many minerals and vitamins in the diet are toxic or even fatal if consumed in too high a dose, for instance. Moreover, "poisons" found in food are often controlled through the judicious use of food processing. Following this example, raw almonds that have not been processed in some way (e.g., roasting, steaming, irradiation) carry a higher concentration of hydrogen cyanide and are also prone to foodborne pathogens like salmonella. Raw almonds were the source of several salmonella outbreaks in 2001 and 2004, in fact; and in 2014 Whole Foods recalled an entire line of raw organic almonds due to elevated levels of cyanide.

Pasteurization, an essential food safety technique that kills pathogens that cause foodborne illness (Chapter 2), also illustrates consumer bias toward foods that are "natural" or "raw." Enthusiasts espouse that raw milk is more salubrious, for example, yet there is copious scientific evidence—including a 2014 review of 81 articles—showing that it carries a far greater risk, despite some minor nutritional benefits (e.g., some healthy bacteria are killed during pasteurization). Indeed, raw milk and dairy products have been shown to carry 14 different types/species of bacteria, three different viruses, and one parasite (*Giardia*), all of which can cause serious sickness. Two large studies are informative. The first collected data between 1993 and 2006, finding that 73 outbreaks in the US were linked to raw milk and cheese versus 48 outbreaks related to pasteurized dairy. These 73 outbreaks caused 4413 cases of foodborne illness, 239 hospitalizations, and 3 deaths. The authors calculated that given the small amount of unpasteurized milk sold in the US, *the risk of outbreak is an astounding 150 times greater or more compared to pasteurized milk.* A more recent study examined outbreaks from 2006 to 2012, finding an increasing number attributed to raw milk each year and that 59% of outbreaks involved at least 1 child under 5 years. (The rise is likely related to weak regulations as more states are allowing the sale of unpasteurized milk.)

Beyond even raw milk is a growing number of "raw food" enthusiasts who tout the health benefits of eating "live" foods, which are more "natural." (A recent culinary encounter of mine featured a "live" lasagna, which was, in effect, a salad. Or so I learned.) In fact, cooking generally enables bioavailability, or the ability of the body to take up a food's valuable nutrients. Cooking may have even been a key to our larger brains, some scientists suggest, as more nutrients and energy became available through heating. Certainly cooking can also destroy nutrients, too, though levels are usually inconsequential, all things considered.

Nevertheless, a healthy halo still surrounds the words "natural" and "raw." A Consumer Reports survey showed that 60% of Americans seek out "natural" foods for perceived healthfulness, for instance. FDA currently allows use of the term on a wide array of processed foods as long as "nothing artificial or synthetic (including all color additives regardless of source) has been included in, or has been added to, a food that would not normally be expected to be in that food." But there is no legal definition—and the guideline says nothing about the nutritional content or other factors of potential interest to consumers. A "natural" granola bar, for instance, may be laden in salt, saturated fat, and sugar. Nature Valley faced a lawsuit over its use of the "n"-word, as have Quaker Oats, General Mills, and smaller brands like Seventh Generation and Honest Co. The suits have arisen in part because "natural" leaves too much room for interpretation among companies, often confusing or misleading consumers about nutritional value. FDA requested public comments in 2016 on using "natural" in food packaging, and clearer regulations may emerge in the future as a result.

As for "clean eating," this phrase started appearing ubiquitously a few years back, and it's a favorite among today's food and health bloggers and celebrities. Others tend to despise it given its converse: "dirty" seems to imply a moral and value judgment about not just the foods but also, perhaps, those who consume them. And many nutritionists remind us that "clean eating" has no scientific meaning and seems to be used simply as a feel-good concept, defined however the user deems best. It certainly *sounds* like a good thing to those seeking health—just like the word "natural"—but it's not a term you'll find used in nutrition science, which is based in biochemistry. "Clean eating" is just another catchphrase, clickbait to drive consumer eyeballs, attention, and sales. (And it certainly doesn't facilitate an informed and nuanced view of food and nutrition.)

More often than not, the clean eating, natural, and raw food concepts hang out together in a junk-science club, providing a false sense of security without being clear about where food is coming from and how it's produced—let alone how it impacts health, society, or the environment. Clean/unclean, raw/cooked, natural/synthetic: these are false dichotomies that obscure far more important nutrition principles critical for health and disease prevention. They also drown out science and create confusion surrounding what healthy eating actually looks like. At worse, food fads like these are dangerous, even fatal, if they come with a serving of foodborne pathogens.

Ignore terms like these, and stick to science when it comes to your health.

What's the difference between "organic" and "conventional"?

"Organic" and "conventional" refer to different sets of farming practices. Conventional agriculture is based on industrial processes and techniques, including synthetic fertilizers and pesticides, intensive tilling, and complex irrigation systems to manage soil and crops; concentrated animal feeding operations (CAFOs, Chapter 12) that often use antibiotics and hormones and minimize (or disregard) animal welfare and well being; and genetic engineering to breed crops and animals in addition to traditional crop breeding. Conventional agriculture is focused on maximizing the yield and efficiency of a single animal or crop, and practices have led to many negative externalities throughout the food system, people to planet.

Organic agriculture grew out of the interest in developing alternative practices that were safer for farmworkers and less harmful to the environment. The FAO/WHO Codex Alimentarius Commission, which puts forth international food standards, defined the practice in 1999:

> Organic agriculture is a holistic production management system which promotes and enhances agro-ecosystem health, including biodiversity, biological cycles, and soil biological activity. It emphasizes the use of management practices in preference to the use of off-farm inputs, taking into account that regional conditions require locally adapted systems. This is accomplished by using, where possible, agronomic, biological, and mechanical methods, as opposed to using synthetic materials, to fulfill any specific function within the system.

FAO does not permit genetic engineering in organic agriculture. Some organic farms include different crops and animals to create an ecosystem that manages pests and protects the soil in lieu of chemicals, though others look no different from a conventional farm, with rows and rows of a single crop (i.e., monoculture). Many countries have certification programs that articulate specific practices that can and can't be used on organic farms and specific guidelines for animal welfare and feed. In the US, certification enables farmers to use a "USDA Organic" label, which often commands a higher price tag than conventional counterparts.

Notably, both conventional and organic agriculture employ pesticides (Chapter 2), the only difference being whether the chemicals are naturally or synthetically derived. Rotenone, for instance, is found in the stems and seeds of some plants and commonly used as a pesticide in organic farming. It is nonselective, which means that it attacks a wide variety of pests, and has been used successfully to kill invasive fish to restore indigenous species in lakes and reservoirs. Perhaps because it is "natural," rotenone was originally assumed to be nontoxic in humans. But a number of studies in both animals and humans have since shown an increased risk of Parkinson's disease with rotenone exposure. Though rotenone is classified as mild compared to many other synthetic pesticides—all pesticides are ranked according to toxicity—this example is included to underscore that just because something is "natural" does not mean that it is inherently safe.

EFSA studied 3090 samples of organic crops across 25 countries in 2009, finding concentrations of eight different prohibited synthetic pesticides—although maximum residue levels for pesticides were still lower on average in organic compared to conventional produce. Pesticide residues on organic produce have likewise been reported in other studies around the world. Why some organic farms have used synthetic pesticides is unknown, though presumably it is to protect the harvest when biopesticides and other organic methods were unsuccessful.

Chemical exposures of any kind can impact health and development, synthetic or natural (think: tobacco exposure during pregnancy). A key finding of the above report and others like it is that pesticide exposure posed no short-term human health risk. Specifically, pesticide residues were detected in both organic and conventional produce, and while concentrations were often higher in conventional produce, they were still lower than the maximum thresholds and not associated with an increased health risk. Special consideration is given to children, who are more susceptible to potential health risks from pesticide exposure due to incomplete immune system development. Yet the conclusions remain the same: the American Academy of Pediatrics and others recommend a diet rich in produce, whether conventional or organic, because the health benefits of consuming vegetables and fruits outweigh any potential unknown risk of pesticide exposure.

There are people who do suffer poor health outcomes due to pesticide exposure, however: farmworkers. Many studies have shown that farmers have a higher risk of neurological, liver, and respiratory diseases as well as type 2 diabetes mellitus (T2DM), some cancers, and cardiovascular diseases (CVD), in addition to Parkinson's. This is the result of chronic exposure to high levels of many different kinds of pesticides, often through skin contact or inhalation during application. Farmers in developing countries face even greater risks (Chapter 2).

Organic enthusiasts often claim such foods are more nutritious than their conventional cousins. There's little reason why a carrot grown using conventional methods should differ significantly in nutrient composition compared to one grown organically: a carrot is a carrot. Yet chemical exposures can influence development of any organism. Thus, numerous studies have compared the nutritional content of organic versus conventional produce. Studies show considerable variability since farming practices vary so widely: What pesticides were used? In what amounts? How often were they applied? And when? Small differences can often be detected for a few nutrients, though they are usually insignificant—and would not lead to meaningful difference in health. Organizations across the board, from WHO to the Environmental Working Group, emphasize the importance of consuming a diet rich in plants, however they're grown: it is far better for your health (and likely no risk at all) to consume copious plant foods for optimal health and disease prevention, whether conventional or organic.

There are various differences beyond chemical usage between organic and conventional techniques that differently impact the environment. For example, organic producers are more likely to practice methods that maintain soil fertility (like crop rotation, low tilling, and use of legume cover crops that return carbon to the soil); reduce fertilizer runoff and subsequent pollution of waterways; promote biodiversity by managing pests and weeds through a diverse set of crops and pollinators, not just chemicals; and others. A meta-analysis of 766 studies found that 327 of 396 showed greater biodiversity on organic compared to conventional farms and that biodiversity contributes to long-term sustainability. There is thus much evidence that, in aggregate, organic agriculture is kinder to the environment.

While part of sustainability is protecting the planet, so is protecting livelihoods through maintaining yield, particularly for subsistence farmers in the developing world. Individual studies reach different conclusions about how organic farming influences crop productivity, which is a critical element of food security. The answer is complex as the state of the soil is pertinent to yield and varies tremendously across a wide range of farming practices: in general, intensive agricultural practices foster lower yields until the soil is restored, irrigated soils without extensive damage foster similar yields, and farming environments with low inputs and natural irrigation foster increased yields. Yields on organic farms may thus differ as a function of prior farming practices, as suggested by FAO, requiring time until soil health returns. (And David R. Montgomery sardonically reminds us in *Scientific American* that "the oft-cited yield gap between conventional and organic farming is smaller than the amount of food we routinely throw away.") Because organic systems generally employ practices that protect the soil and are less destructive to natural ecosystems, they tend to be more sustainable than conventional agriculture. Still, sustainability is ultimately dependent on the use of fossil fuels throughout the farming system, and neither organic nor conventional systems will be truly sustainable until renewable and alternative energy sources are used throughout agriculture.

Is "eating local" important for human health and the environment?

Local food is a way of life for many in the developing world. Yet in the US and other high-income countries, "eating local" has become a trendy phrase found everywhere from fine dining to fast food, university campuses to workplace cafeterias. Those committed to eating local often refer to themselves as "locavores" and are focused on food that has not traveled a long distance to market, thereby reducing "food miles." Though some use a 100-mile radius from farm to fork as a guidepost, there is no scientific consensus among agricultural organizations that defines local based on geographic distance between production and consumption. Rather, "local" is a function of marketing arrangements, according to the US Department of Agriculture (USDA).

In the Western construct, eating local has numerous benefits, including tasting the best food around, sustaining the businesses of local farmers, supporting regional food systems, preserving common land and its biodiversity, and building a community that cares about food. These are excellent reasons to eat local—if you're in a place where farmers' markets are accessible, affordable, and convenient.

Yet substantial folklore surrounds "eating local," often touted affectionately and adamantly by farmers market aficionados. The first myth regards nutritional composition. Whereas the soil can significantly impact a plant's concentration of certain minerals (like selenium) and species genotype also matters, a crop is what it is. All apples, for example, provide vitamin C, fiber, water, and a host of phytochemicals (Chapter 7). But how it is picked, stored, and transported all impact nutrient content more significantly than where it was grown. For instance, a carrot picked at its peak of ripeness, flash-frozen on site, stored in your freezer, then steamed briefly for your supper can have significantly higher beta-carotene than a carrot picked a few days (or weeks or months) prior, transported by truck, sat at the local market in the heat, brought home, and left in your fridge until you ate it who-knows-when.

The second myth is that local is more sustainable. Thinking about seafood in particular, many wild-caught, local species have been overfished to the point of extinction, and those caught from nearby streams and lakes carry a higher risk of contamination from mercury and other toxins. How seafood is caught matters as some methods lead to substantial by-catch, thus contributing to food waste (Chapter 2). For these reasons, wild-caught, nonlocal species may be the most sustainable choice, or perhaps farmed seafood, depending on how the fish are raised (Chapter 13). The factors influencing seafood sustainability are complex and further vary by species and geography—and stocks change as protected species rebound and fisheries are replenished. Sustainable seafood recommendations vary over time, and there are many consumer apps and sources online to guide informed decision-making. As with plants and other animals, seafood sustainability is primarily a function of production practices, not proximity to home.

The third myth touts that eating local is the best dietary choice for the environment. It is certainly true that local foods have fewer "food miles," as they've traveled a shorter distance from farm to table than those traversing the country, or even globe. But that doesn't necessarily mean your local apple has a smaller carbon footprint than one imported. Economies of scale matter, as does mode of transport: millions of apples arriving by ship often have a smaller carbon footprint per unit than thousands traveling by truck. Moreover, food production contributes 83% of greenhouse gas emissions (GHGe) compared to just 11% for food transportation. Indeed, production impacts on climate are larger than *all* post–farm gate emissions (transport, retail, waste) for almost all foods, and animal foods create the most GHGe by far (Chapter 12). The science is clear: the best dietary choice for the environment is to eat less meat, wherever you buy it, not eat local. Those consuming an almost exclusively plant-based diet from fresh foods, like vegans, are a potential exception, depending on the crop.

An additional myth asserts that local food is safer. The life cycle chain from farm to fork is often shorter and more transparent within local systems, which can help to quickly identify sources of foodborne illness. Yet there are no conclusive data that local food is any safer, and smaller systems can lack the quality control and practices of larger counterparts. Local wares sitting at a farmers' market in hot temperatures are also a breeding ground for bacteria if improperly stored—and many purveyors favor raw milk and juices, which are substantially less safe than those pasteurized.

A final myth is that eating local is less expensive. Great deals can abound at farmers' markets, especially when buying in bulk. But prices for conventional produce are generally comparable to or higher than those in your average supermarket—and local organic produce can be downright exorbitant. Happily, many markets now participate in food assistance programs to increase affordability to lower-income individuals. Furthermore, local foods are increasingly available at mainstream supermarkets, often leading to more attractive prices and greater accessibility that make it easier for eaters of all incomes to support local food systems and all the good things they represent.

While eating local will doubtless play a role in future food systems, it is not a panacea for today's complex food and nutrition problems in a global food supply.

OMG GMO!? Why is food genetically engineered?

Do you know someone with diabetes who needs insulin? Chances are it was synthesized using genetic engineering (GE), like many other life-saving medicines. Love cheese? Rennet is a collection of enzymes used in traditional cheesemaking produced by ruminants, usually calves—but the majority is now synthesized animal-free using GE.

Plants or animals in which genes have been altered using molecular biology and recombinant DNA techniques rather than conventional breeding are colloquially referred to as genetically modified organisms (GMOs), or, alternatively, GE or "biotech" crops. GE allows direct and specific changes to a plant's DNA, ribonucleic acid (RNA), or proteins to create, express, or repress a trait rather than achieve the same end through conventional cross-breeding. In "transgenic" species, which receive the most media and consumer attention, genes from a different species are inserted. Yet adding a gene from the same species (cisgenic) and modifying a gene within the same species (such as turning it on or off) are also examples of GE (see Chapter 3). In 2017, 11 biotech foods were commercially available in the US: corn, soybeans, cotton, canola, alfalfa, and sugar beet (for insect and/or herbicide resistance); papaya and squash (virus resistance); apple (browning resistance); potato (blight resistance); and salmon (faster growth).

GE crops have been produced since the early 1990s and have been the subject of thousands of scientific investigations. A gargantuan review of 1738 studies between 2002 and 2012 examined impacts on such factors as traceability, biodiversity, safety, and gene flow (into wild species, for example), finding no significant health or environmental hazards. And a 2014 meta-analysis of 147 studies found that GE crops reduced chemical pesticide use by 37%, increased crop yields by 22%, and increased farmer profits by 68%. In 2016, a National Academies of Sciences, Engineering, and Medicine report concluded, "While recognizing the inherent difficulty of detecting subtle or long-term effects in health or the environment, the study committee found no substantiated evidence of a difference in risks to human health between currently commercialized genetically engineered (GE) crops and conventionally bred crops, nor did it find conclusive cause-and-effect evidence of environmental problems from the GE crops." These reports are consistent with those from governmental and nongovernmental agencies around the world.[2]

Even so, many eaters oppose the use of GMOs—though they've been consuming foods made with them for years with no (observed) ill effects. While conversations related to food politics and ethics are vital—like who owns the technology, how it is used, who benefits, who doesn't, and why—conflation with science has limited, and is still limiting, the use of a potentially life- and planet-saving technology. Moreover, GMO anti-science distracts eaters from critical nutrition and environmental issues: focusing on the overall composition of the diet and the planetary consequences of food production, whether for weight loss, disease prevention, longevity, or sustainability, will have a far greater impact on individual lives and our collective society.

Is "grass-fed" beef healthier and more sustainable than "grain-fed"?

There is both misinformation and oversimplification regarding the differences between "grass-fed" and "grain-fed" beef. In fact, all cows begin grazing in pasture, which is why deforestation is a major driver of meat production regardless of system. The key difference is that grain-fed cows are usually moved into concentrated animal feeding operations (CAFOs) and fed grain-based diets until slaughter, while grass-fed cattle remain on pasture; they are thus technically referred to as "grass-finished." Grain-fed cattle, common in conventional agriculture, are more "efficient" because they reach market weight sooner—due to a diet high in calories and starch and a lack of physical activity—and thus require less land and fewer resources. Yet, while grass-finished cattle do produce more waste and methane as a function of living longer, they also consume fewer antibiotics due to better living conditions. They may also be raised on farms that include plants and animals, providing benefits to natural ecosystems.

For example, one study showed that conventional systems required 56% of the animals, 25% of the water, 55% of the land, and 71% of the fossil fuel compared to grass-finished systems, thereby producing a smaller overall carbon footprint per unit of beef. However, the study did not consider variables like antibiotic resistance, animal welfare, and worker safety and health, each of which adds expenses to the environment and society. It also did not assess the true water cost differences: conventional cattle consume less water during their shorter lives, but other costs are higher, like watering pasture and feed crops. Thirsty crops like corn require irrigation, for instance, whereas grass-finished cattle consume grass, forage, and fodder that are generally rain-fed. Finally, the study did not examine differences in carbon sequestration (i.e., carbon moves from the atmosphere to soil to crops to animal and back to the atmosphere through respiration), which has been found to decrease the carbon footprint of grass-fed cattle in several studies in the US, UK, and Ireland.

There are also nutritional differences between grass-finished and grain-fed cattle, an example of "you are what you eat eats." The biggest difference is fat composition: corn is high in omega-6 fatty acids like linoleic acid, whereas grass provides some plant-based omega-3 fatty acids (Chapter 8). As many Western diets are especially low in omega-3 fatty acids, grass-fed beef makes a larger contribution to intake relative to grain-fed beef. Yet quantities are incomparable to the amounts in seafood (Chapter 13). Grass-fed beef is also higher in CLA (i.e., conjugated linoleic acid) and has higher beta-carotene and alpha-tocopherol (precursors to vitamin A and vitamin E, respectively); other small micronutrient differences may occur due to nutrient variability in feed and soil.

Still, many eaters prefer the fatty, marbled meat from grain-fed beef compared to the leaner, gamier flavor from grass-finished. Fortunately, the social acceptability of CAFO beef has decreased: one study found that consumers were less willing to pay for grain-fed beef when educated about the use of growth-enhancing technologies like antibiotics. Therefore, greater awareness may help shift eating habits in a more sustainable direction.

How does "wild-caught" salmon compare to "farmed"?

All salmon provide critical omega-3 fatty acids eicosapentaenoic acid (EPA) and docosahexaenoic acid (DHA) (Chapter 8), whether farmed or wild-caught. Wild salmon are carnivorous and feed mainly on krill and shrimp, which are rich in the orange-hued carotenoid astaxanthin. Farmed salmon don't eat these foods; hence, their flesh is gray, then colored using manufactured astaxanthin (for consumer preference purposes). Nutrient composition further varies depending on how the fish are farmed (Chapter 13). Many aquaculture systems initially used smaller fish, marine-based fishmeal, and fish oil to mimic natural diets, though feed today is often plant-based agricultural byproducts like rapeseed, corn, soybeans, rice, and wheat. (Some farms also include ground-up feathers, yeast, soybeans, and chicken fat in their feed.) Carbohydrate-based diets are higher in omega-6 fatty acids and alter the fat composition of the fish.

Wild salmon are perceived as being more nutritious than farmed, specifically regarding their lower fat and purportedly higher EPA and DHA content. Wild salmon do swim far greater distances—they are not raised in a pen—and thus tend to be leaner. EPA and DHA (omega-3) levels in wild fish vary based on factors like age, sex, species, season, reproductive status, and food availability. Wild salmon are often caught during spawning and migration, for example, leading to lower overall fat and omega-3 content compared to farmed salmon. Fillet fat of farmed Norwegian salmon was 12% on average in one study, for instance, almost double that in wild counterparts. Farmed salmon in the US were also generally higher in total fat compared to wild-caught. Overall, the scientific consensus is that farmed salmon is generally higher in EPA and DHA compared to wild, on average, in part as a function of its overall higher fat content, and that concentration varies by feed. Farmed salmon fed fish oil and fish byproducts have a higher concentration of EPA and DHA compared to those fed diets based on plants or other foods, notably.[3] Importantly, salmon from any source, wild or farmed, has more EPA and DHA than most other fish species—and any other terrestrial animal, including grass-fed beef.

Similar investigations have compared the nutrition profile of other wild and farmed species, with mixed results for reasons discussed. Farmed bass, cod, and trout have as much or more EPA and DHA compared to wild-caught in many high-income nations. (Farmed catfish and crawfish had lower EPA and DHA compared to wild, although these species are not good sources of omega-3 fatty acids regardless.) Conversely, a study in Bangladesh summed intakes of 63 different fish species consumed in more than 5000 households and compared nutrient intakes among wild-caught and farmed variants. Wild-caught fish made a larger contribution to iron, zinc, calcium, vitamin A, and vitamin B_{12} intakes among participants. These results are perhaps attributable to fish farming in these cases being subsistence aquaculture, leading to considerable differences in the nutrient quality of feed.

A final comparison of wild and farmed seafood regards potential contamination as many wild species have been exposed to persistent organic pollutants like mercury. The 2015 Scientific Advisory Committee of the Dietary Guidelines for Americans examined one international seafood composition database and four country-specific databases (Japan, France, Norway, US). The committee concluded that mercury and dioxin (and polychlorinated biphenyl, or PCB) differences between wild and farmed seafood were not appreciably different except for Pacific wild salmon, which had significantly lower levels of dioxins.

The significant differences between farmed and wild species are not about nutrient content or contamination but, rather, about whether the methods by which they were produced—or caught—were environmentally sustainable and socially conscious. Capture fisheries and aquaculture methods differ widely across farm and ocean, depending on the country of origin. Practices evolve, as demonstrated in salmon farming, while wild stocks can change in response to fishing regulations (Chapter 13). Keeping track of whether the wild or farmed variant of a given species is most sustainable at any one time is tough. Organizations dedicated to protecting oceans and waterways (e.g., Monterey Bay Aquarium, Blue Ocean Institute, National Geographic) provide accurate and up-to-date information on which seafood is most sustainable, and consulting their websites or downloading their apps can inform sustainable and healthy seafood choices.

Is sugar addictive?

Our highly palatable food environment combined with our innate preference for sweet foods (Chapter 5) has led many to question whether sugar is addictive. Sugar activates pleasure centers in the brain in a similar fashion to drugs. And some experiments in animals have shown that neurobiological changes in the brain following sugar consumption are similar to drug addiction. For example, Lenoir and colleagues tested how rats responded to sugar and saccharin solutions versus cocaine when offered as a reward. They found that 94% of animals preferred sugar, stimulating a barrage of "Sugar is more addictive than cocaine!" headlines.[4] This and other animal studies also show tolerance and withdrawal symptoms to sugar that are suggestive of addiction.

Research in humans is equivocal, however. Sugar is certainly habit-forming, and too much of it carries risks of obesity, heart disease, and T2DM (Chapter 8). But a 2016 review found little evidence that sugar shares the same neurochemical properties as drugs like cocaine. Moreover, effects in animals often result from experimental conditions that don't apply to humans, like total sugar deprivation and/or highly concentrated solutions that drive consumption. Nor is our biology the same. The authors thus concluded that "the science of sugar addiction at present is not compelling." Likewise, the American Psychiatric Association does not recognize sugar addiction.

Whether sugar is addictive remains an active research area. Physician Robert Lustig, for instance, suggests that sugar, salt, and caffeine together—the hallmarks of many a fast food meal— may individually or in concert fuel overeating and food addiction, noting that some obese individuals show impaired resistance to appetite and reward signals in the brain. He adds that a cycle of stress and dieting may sensitize reward centers and, when combined with constant cues to consume palatable foods, "may trigger overeating." He concludes that fast food may be a "potentially addictive substance that is most likely to create dependence in vulnerable populations."

The current scientific consensus is that sugar does not appear to be addictive in humans, though knowledge will certainly advance and may inform dietary behavior (change) in the future, particularly in those with specific circumstances or genes. Yet whether or not sugar is "addictive" as such is, for most people, way beside the point: we eat too much sugar because it's innate, it's delectable, and it's everywhere we look. And change is possible (Chapter 17)—without rehab.

What are "good bacteria," and how are they related to "probiotics," "prebiotics," and the "microbiome"?

There are about 30–37.2 trillion human cells in the body, the majority (84%) of which are red blood cells. And there are some 39 trillion bacterial cells on average, generally ranging from 30 to 50 trillion. Bacteria are just one kind of nonhuman cell that resides in our bodies, which also includes a host of other microorganisms like fungi and viruses. All together, microorganisms (or microbes) outnumber human cells by at least 3 to 1, based on newer estimates from a 2016 study, or perhaps as much as 10 to 1. They live throughout the body and on its surface and constitute what is known as the human microbiome. About 90–95% live in the gut, particularly the colon, where their metabolic activity influences systems and organs throughout the body.

While some microbes are pathogenic, or cause disease, the majority live harmoniously with our own human cells. Why some microbes end up wreaking havoc in some people but not others is a big part of untangling how the microbiome impacts health. To that end, the Human Microbiome Project of the National Institutes of Health began mapping the DNA of microbes found in humans in 2007. Scientists discovered more than 10 000 distinct species that, in aggregate, coded around 8 million proteins—dwarfing our own human genome, which carries about 22 000 protein-coding genes.

Copious factors shape the composition of the human microbiome, which can vary profoundly across humans depending on such variables as geographic location, diet, and overall state of health. Sickness impacts the microbiome, which is further disrupted if the patient is taking antibiotics, which kill pathogenic and healthy bacteria alike. Studies have shown that the microbiome is robust and will rebound, though its composition may vary. (It is for this reason that taking antibiotics without clear reason is ill-advised.)

A fascinating study observed striking differences between the microbes of Hadza hunter–gatherers in Tanzania and Italians in Bologna. The Hadza, whose meals fluctuate with the wet and dry seasons and food availability—and who consume hundreds more distinct species of foods compared to consumers of Western diets— also showed corresponding shifts in gut bacteria. In contrast, the Italians' microbiome was stable and lacked seasonal variability, a reflection of Western diets that provide food of any kind, at any time. Further comparison to a host of other groups around the world (like those living in American cities or Amazon rainforest villages) showed similar results: seasonal eaters showed a wider variety in the gut microbiome and more fluctuations compared to those consuming Western diets. And many of the gut microbes were rare and *only* occurred in traditional societies.

While extreme variability of the human microbiome across the world is perhaps unsurprising, there are nonetheless significant differences observed even among those in similar places. Generally speaking, there are two types of foods that influence the gut microbiome. *Probiotics* are live microorganisms consumed in the diet, like the bacterial strains *Streptococcus thermophilus* and *Lactobacillus bulgaricus* commonly found in yogurt (Chapter 12). Other fermented foods contain probiotics, including kimchi, a traditional Korean vegetable dish often made with lactic acid bacteria, and kombucha, a sweet tea made with both bacteria and yeast (Chapter 14). *Prebiotics* are not live microorganisms but, rather, feed beneficial ("good") microbes; they include some fibers and refined starches that are fermented by gut bacteria. ("Synbiotics" refers to foods or meals containing both probiotics and prebiotics.) Both probiotics and prebiotics increase the proportion of good bacteria in the gut and evoke positive health effects. They are especially important when the gut microbiota is out of balance, perhaps due to a health condition.

Unraveling the mysteries of the "optimal" microbiome will take many decades, including what precisely it comprises and how it can be restored when disrupted. Still, nutrition research is increasingly showing the valuable effects of probiotics and prebiotics on a range of gut conditions, like inflammatory bowel disease and irritable bowel syndrome. And their role in the immune system likely influences allergic and autoimmune diseases as well. There are also some studies suggesting that the microbiome appears important for chronic diseases like obesity and T2DM, as well as a range of neuropsychiatric diseases, though more research is needed.

Why is breastfeeding important?

WHO's Convention on the Rights of the Child asserts that every kid has the right to good nutrition—and good nutrition begins at the breast. There is an adage among nutritionists that "breast is best" when it comes to feeding your newborn; and, unlike so many other diet axioms out there, this one is actually true. The reasons are simple and intuitive: breast milk contains everything new-to-the-world mammals need nutritionally to begin their healthiest lives.

Breast milk has about 171 calories per cup (i.e., 70 calories per 100 g), and its nutrient composition changes over time to meet the different needs of the rapidly growing newborn. The first liquid to come from a mother's breast, colostrum, is high in growth factors and rich in immune system building chemicals (like immunoglobulins) that fight infection. Over time, varying from a few days to a couple of weeks, the lactose composition of the milk increases ("transitional milk") and the mineral composition shifts to include more potassium and calcium and less sodium, chloride, and magnesium. It also contains unique oligosaccharides (Chapter 8), prebiotics that feed healthy gut bacteria like *Bifidobacterium infantis*. And newer research is finding that breast milk is also a rich source of probiotics, including more than 700 species of microbes that further contribute to the developing gut microbiome. The "fully mature" breast milk is produced by the time a baby reaches 4–6 weeks, and the basic composition remains stable throughout breastfeeding.[5]

Maternal diet influences the composition of breast milk, especially its fat and micronutrient (e.g., vitamins A, B_1, B_2, B_6, B_{12}, and D as well as iodine) concentrations. The omega-3 fatty acid DHA is particularly variable since this essential fatty acid (Chapter 7) must be obtained from the diet. DHA is critical for brain and visual development, but studies have shown that composition is low among women consuming limited amounts of seafood, the primary source. This is why many organizations recommend that breastfeeding women consume 2–3 servings of seafood weekly. Though contamination of fish by mercury and other toxins scared pregnant and nursing women into cutting back on seafood several years ago, research remains clear that the benefits of DHA to growing fetuses and infants override the risks (Chapter 13). DHA may also be obtained through a nutritional supplement, and vegan alternatives made from algae are also available.

The impacts of breastfeeding on child health are so profound that UNICEF calls it a "miracle investment . . . the closest thing the world has to a magic bullet for child survival." Much of this is because of the immune-boosting compounds breast milk provides, which means children who breastfeed are less susceptible to life-threatening infections like pneumonia and diarrhea; these are extremely common among children in the developing world. Breast milk also contains a wide range of bioactive components (e.g., growth factors, hormones) critical for building healthy organs and systems. Breast milk components also have epigenetic effects, which fine-tune genetic expression in infants and can impact health and disease risk throughout life.

Exclusively breastfed children are in fact 14 times more likely to survive than non-breastfed children—and have been found to have higher intelligence on average. A 2016 study that included 28 systematic reviews and meta-analyses estimated that more than 823 000 deaths in children under age 5 could be prevented if breastfeeding were universally adopted. Importantly, HIV^+ mothers are now able to breastfeed due to advances in antiretroviral drugs. Moms benefit too: breastfeeding reduces the risk of post-partum hemorrhage and produces amenorrhea (loss of periods) that reduces pregnancy risk, critical for healthy child spacing.

More recent research has examined longer-term effects in childhood and beyond, including asthma, food allergies, T2DM, and obesity. Additional studies have also investigated associations with reproductive cancers in mothers as well as osteoporosis, depression, post-partum weight loss, and others. Support for most of these relationships is equivocal, though there is strong evidence of a 26% reduced risk of breast cancer among women who breastfed exclusively.

In addition to the nutritional benefits of breastfeeding, the shared experience facilitates mother–baby bonding, providing social and emotional benefits to both. Breast milk is also free of cost, critically important among mothers with limited income. Finally, breast milk is often the safest food for infants as most infant formula requires a clean and ample water supply and/or refrigeration. For all of these reasons and more, WHO recommends that infants are breastfed exclusively for at least 6 months; breastfeeding should start within a few hours of birth for maximal protection. Yet only 43% of infants 0–6 months globally are exclusively breastfed, with a smaller percentage (37%) in low- and middle-income countries. Challenges include building awareness about breastfeeding's importance; strengthening government policies and programs that support breastfeeding, especially in the developing world; and developing safe spaces for women to breastfeed in public, as well as in the workplace. One of WHO's global goals is to increase those exclusively breastfed to at least 50% by 2025.

How does infant formula compare to breast milk?

Despite the abundant benefits breastfeeding brings to both baby and mother, there are some for whom breastfeeding is simply not possible. The act is far more difficult than new mothers are led to believe, often requiring substantial support for success—and prohibitive policies shaming breastfeeding create barriers. Health conditions compromising milk production and composition may also play a role. Social and economic pressures can lead women to truncate breastfeeding or forgo it completely. In addition, breastfeeding remains shrouded in social mores associated with wealth and class, which still shape women's choices in some countries. Finally, advertising practices and provision of free formula in hospitals by powerful food marketers often undermine breastfeeding messages.

For all of these reasons and others, women have for generations sought alternatives to breast milk from prehistory to present.[6] In the 19th century, advances in science and technology dovetailed with a greater need to provide alternatives to breastfeeding, culminating in the first commercial infant formula created in 1867 by chemist Justus von Leibig. His powder mixture was combined with cow's milk, although later products of his (and others) included evaporated milk that could be mixed with water (1874). A glass baby bottle and rubber teats had been patented in 1845, enabling easier feeding compared to spoons and horns used previously. By 1883, there were 27 different brands (!) of formula available.

During the following century, there was much trial and error in creating suitable infant formula, but results were limited by incomplete knowledge of breast milk's chief components. Scientific advances led to a greater understanding of both breast milk and the nutritional needs (e.g., vitamins and minerals) of growing babies. As well, better methods for synthesizing artificial alternatives were created, enabling production of safe, shelf-stable infant formula. Today's formula is the closest thing nutritionally to breast milk, now including the essential omega-3 fatty acid DHA for infant development. Formula is age-specific, too, reflecting the change from colostrum to transitional to mature breast milk. Still, formula can only be as good as current scientific knowledge, which is always evolving; and there is no substitute for the individualized immune protection and microbes that come from maternal milk: breast will always be best, an "exquisite personalized medicine" that benefits both child and mother in ways we still do not fully appreciate.

5

DIETS AND FOOD ENVIRONMENTS TODAY

WHY WE EAT THE WAY WE DO

What are the influencers and major drivers of eating behavior and food choices in today's world?

For millions of years during the course of evolution, the human diet was driven simply by hunger and accessibility. As civilizations developed, money also became a factor in who could eat. Still today, hunger and cost are the major factors driving food behavior, particularly for those with limited income. On average, low-income nations spend a higher percentage of their income on food, whereas high- and middle-income nations spend a lower percentage. The US Department of Agriculture (USDA) collects information on average food expenditures across almost 90 countries around the world. In 2014, the US spent the smallest proportion of income on food annually (6.6%), while Nigeria spent the largest (56.6%); absolute food expenditures translated to $USD per capita were highest in Norway ($4413, or 12.3% of income) and lowest in India ($302, 30.2% of income).

Individuals living in regions with abundant food and adequate financial resources have the luxury of creating a diet based on biological (e.g., taste), social (e.g., family, peer, community), psycho-emotional (e.g., stress, mood), cognitive (e.g., beliefs, education), and economic (e.g., cost, price) factors. The larger agri-food system and overall food environment also determine what is available and accessible. For many, spiritual traditions play a vital role, like in Hinduism (vegetarian), Judaism (kosher), and Islam (no alcohol). All of these different influences on eating behavior intertwine, often with distinct local, regional, and national flair, to create a rich variety of food cultures and practices around the world.

Despite the myriad factors that shape overall eating behavior, the subject of the current chapter, study after study shows that taste takes the cake when it comes to making everyday food choices. Cost is the second biggest variable. In the US, for example, the International Food Information Council (IFIC) surveyed the value Americans placed on the roles of taste, cost, healthfulness, convenience, and sustainability on food choice, ranked on a scale of 1 (no impact) to 5 (great impact). In 2015, 83% ranked taste as having an impact of 4 or 5, followed by cost (68%), healthfulness (60%), and convenience (52%). IFIC only began measuring the impact of sustainability on food choices in 2011, when 52% ranked it as a 4 or 5, though this percentage dropped significantly to 35% in 2015. The degree to which such factors play a role depends on things like income, gender, and age. Convenience and price were valued more by younger participants, while taste and healthfulness were ranked higher among those with greater income. Women, who are more likely to purchase food for their families, ranked healthfulness, cost, and sustainability more strongly than men.

Understanding the basic drivers of food choice is critical to the success of programs aimed at dietary behavior change and positive health outcomes, like losing weight or managing type 2 diabetes mellitus (T2DM). Knowing what people like and eat, and how often, is also critical for successful nutrification programs (Chapter 6). Marketers are as keen to understand eating behavior as health professionals since it informs new product development and drives product sales on busy supermarket shelves. In fact, much food choice research comes not from social scientists but from the food industry—which tends to have far more money and influence to shape food choices, for better and worse.

What exactly is taste, and why does it differ across person and place?

Tasting food is one of life's simplest, most sensual pleasures. When an aroma hits our nose, we may salivate in anticipation of things to come. And taste can evoke memories of experiences from decades past, pleasant or unpleasant. Biologically speaking, taste is a "chemical detection system" that recognizes nutrients, like sugar, and poisons, like cyanide. It was once thought that there were only four basic tastes—sweet, sour, salty, bitter—each located in separate places on the tongue. Scientists now recognize five distinct tastes. The fifth, umami (savory), was discovered by Japanese researchers in 1910. Researchers are currently investigating whether there are receptors for fatty, alkaline, metallic, and water-like tastes, too. Interestingly, Indian Ayurvedic philosophy recognizes six tastes: sweet, sour, salty, bitter, pungent, and astringent. Our understanding of what and how we taste will, like all things scientific, continue to evolve.

Taste is a multi-organ process, resulting in a wide array of sensations. The tongue is the most obvious. Its bumpy appearance is due to several different kinds of papillae, where taste buds live, and each taste bud has around 10–100 taste cells. The nose is also key as smell stimulates nasal nerve fibers that carry information to the brain. (Hence, those suffering from smell impairment, hyposmia, have a reduced ability to smell and taste food). Newer studies indicate that the oral cavity and gastrointestinal system also participate in taste perception, with their own properties that send information about taste to the brain.

The tongue, which has 2000–4000 taste buds on average, is able to sense each of the five tastes, despite earlier beliefs espousing that certain tastes were experienced in different places. Bitter perception is particularly potent at the back of the tongue, a last stop before potentially toxic substances are ingested. Indeed, scientists believe the ability to recognize foods as bitter evolved as a survival mechanism as plants with such flavors are often poisonous. Sweet-tasting foods have the opposite effect: our bodies like the sensation, and we often want more. Humans innately prefer sweet foods, with copious studies showing these proclivities in newborns. (Sweet often signifies readily available glucose, creating a positive feedback loop in evolving humans that such foods were nutritious and energy-giving.) Newer hypotheses suggest that the ratio of sweet to bitter creates a signal that shaped eating behavior.

Like all things, taste varies from person to person. Some may remember taking a test in a biology class in which a small, bitter-tasting disc is placed on the tongue (or some variation of this experiment). Reactions vary, producing a bell curve of tasting intensity, with those at the tail end—who tend to make an "ewww" face and spit out the disc—being "supertasters." Basic research studies have shown that genetic differences (such as variation in *TASR38*, a bitter taste receptor gene) are responsible. As a result, supertasters often prefer less flavorful food: their ability to perceive taste is already genetically enhanced, as it were. Those with less sensitive taste buds are more likely to enjoy bold flavors since they need a bigger kick, simply speaking, to ignite their taste buds.

Independent of genetic variation, children are better able to perceive both bitter and sweet tastes, harkening again to the evolutionary advantage of allowing time to learn which foods are nutritious and which are fatal. Additional taste buds in places like the lips and hard palate enable amplified perception in childhood, as does increased expression of taste genes. There is indeed a biological basis for kids hating bitter-tasting veggies and loving all things sugary. Yet we lose this heightened sensitivity to bitter and sweet tastes during adolescence, likely because this functionality is no longer necessary once experience is acquired.

Despite biology, taste is not fixed; preferences are an interaction between genes and environment throughout life. Proclivities begin in utero, shaped by what mothers consume during gestation. (Prenatal nutrition shapes a great deal of biological and metabolic activity throughout life, it turns out, depending not only on what kind of foods mothers eat but also how much, including such things as taste preferences as well as allergenicity and fat storage.) Infant and early childhood dietary exposures—nutritional epidemiology speak for what we ate and drank as kids—then interact with so-called fetal programming to shape young palates. Cultural and traditional food behaviors next begin to emerge: Japanese tots begin a diet of white rice, fish, and tofu; Mexican toddlers start enjoying tortillas, beans, and plantains; and Indian kids indulge in spicy curries. Many American and European children grow up with milder flavors at mealtimes, depending on ancestry, yet may discover spicier foods as adults, a result of repeated exposure and positive learning experiences.[1]

Despite learned eating behaviors that are shaped in early childhood and biological differences, like whether one is a supertaster, taste preferences can be modified throughout the life course due to neuroplasticity, which refers to our brain's ability to continue changing even as we age: there is far more flexibility in our (food) behaviors than most think. This is terrific news for adventurous eaters who want to expand their dinner repertoire—it's a big, delicious world out there!—but it's tremendous news for those hoping to ditch poor food habits to create a healthier diet. Just like kids gradually learn to like nutritious foods, so, too, can adults readjust their palate. Many who switch from refined grain foods like white bread and white rice to whole grain variants, for instance, gradually learn to prefer the nutty flavors and toothsome textures. Repeated exposure—and a willingness to change—is the key (Chapter 17).

How does the foodscape shape how we eat?

External factors that impact eating behavior are referred to collectively as the "food environment," or "foodscape." The foodscape can be further divided into macro- and microenvironmental factors, like location, offerings, and price as well as laws, regulations, taxes, and subsidies that shape the agri-food industry.

During the past century, ever more places and ever more products have arisen to feed us whenever and wherever we choose. Eating options even include convenience stores, now with expanded grocery aisles stocked with supermarket staples alongside an overabundance of snack foods and beverages that challenge even the most disciplined eater simply going in to buy a tube of toothpaste. (I'm talking about myself here.) The ubiquity of ultra-processed, high-sugar, energy-dense, nutrient-poor, and inexpensively priced victuals combined with constant cues to consume creates an "obesogenic" food environment, a term coined by scientists Garry Egger and Boyd Swinborn, who call obesity a "normal physiology within a pathological environment."

But is focusing on foodscape factors enough? For example, are neighborhoods lacking supermarkets selling nutritious foods but booming with convenience stores and fast food outlets—"food deserts" or "food swamps," depending on perspective—associated with a higher prevalence of obesity and T2DM? And what about "food mirages," which thrive with pricey specialty and high-end supermarkets but lack affordable grocery stores? These relationships are complex for numerous reasons, including the difficulty in studying the complete food system while accounting for other major contributors to dietary behavior. But careful research indicates that socioeconomic status (SES) is a major driver: income and education shape food choices, not the landscape of food offerings per se. Most people buy groceries at supermarkets, for instance, whether higher income (91%) or lower income (87%), though travel time may differ. Indeed, a fascinating study showed that poorer nutritional choices were still made by lower-SES individuals when supermarkets were added to food deserts, or if families moved to areas with more supermarkets.

Given that a healthy diet can be constructed on lower incomes, as has been demonstrated in a number of studies, poorer food choices could thus reflect a lack of nutrition knowledge. On the other hand, proximity to food swamps replete with fast food joints and corner stores does show an association with unhealthy eating and obesity. Therefore, while lack of knowledge may play some role, it is more likely that such food outlets hit the big three factors influencing food decisions: taste, cost, and convenience. High-stress lifestyles on limited incomes may increase their attractiveness because food is often cheaper per calorie. And lower-SES families may, understandably, place a higher priority on concerns like safety, violence, and food security rather than nutrition.

Studies that consider both individual and environmental factors on eating behavior and obesity in particular are needed, as doubtless some individuals are more vulnerable to external cues from the foodscape than others. We will better appreciate this phenomenon the more we understand the different types of obesity in light of genetic susceptibility that impacts both food preferences and energy balance.

Does food advertising impact diet?

Food advertising is particularly potent in rousing our palates and stimulating demand. According to the American Psychological Association (APA) Task Force on Advertising and Children, kids 8–18 years old spend about 44 hours weekly looking at screens—computer, television, gaming, and the like—and are exposed to approximately 40 000 ads per year, many of them for food.[2] Though measuring food advertising in association with health outcomes like body weight is fraught with methodological difficulties, it has become increasingly clear that the practice is contributing to America's obesity crisis. The APA notes in its report that, because of insufficient cognitive and emotional development, marketing to children is no less than "inherently exploitative."

In response to the substantial body of evidence, the US Federal Trade Commission (FTC) examined the extent and scope of food advertising to youth. The FTC found that 44 major food and beverage marketers spent $2.1 billion marketing food to kids in 2006. The Council of Better Business Bureaus then launched the Children's Food and Beverage Advertising Initiative to self-regulate the industry, and FTC conducted a follow-up among the same companies in 2009 to measure progress. Total spending had dropped to $1.79 billion, mainly due to a 19.5% reduction in television advertising; but the amount of money spent on (less expensive) digital methods increased 50%. Thus, the report concluded that "[t]he overall picture . . . did not significantly change." It also noted that the media and entertainment industry had not curtailed its own advertising (e.g., product placements in children's programming and movies) but for a few exceptions: Disney, for instance, committed to apply nutrition standards to ads in children's programs.

Of course, if the foods being marketed to kids were healthful, then advertising could play a positive role. However, advertising often peddles kid-friendly favorites like sugar-sweetened goodies (e.g., beverages, cereals, yogurts, snacks, candy, frozen desserts), ultra-processed foods high in sodium (e.g., canned soups), and high-calorie fast food. The 2009 data showed that modest improvements had been made, especially in reduced marketing of sugar-sweetened beverages to children (but not teenagers); marketers were able to increase "nutrients to encourage" but had a harder time reducing "nutrients to limit." A classic example is breakfast cereals that are fortified with vitamins and minerals or whole grains but still include a tremendous amount of sugar.

How have cooking and dining changed in the 21st century?

The majority of the world's population still cooks and sups in their own kitchens, often with food from local supermarkets, but cooking is becoming a lost art in many high-income countries. In the US, the NPD Group found that less than 60% of dinners eaten at home were actually cooked at home, down from almost 75% in 1984. (And "home" often reflects takeout or prepared meals from supermarkets, not cooking.) The time spent in meal preparation also dropped dramatically. The Harris Poll reported that 41% of adults cook 5 or more times weekly, 29% cook 3–4 times weekly, 19% cook 1–2 times weekly, and 11% "rarely" or "never" cook at home. Among other reasons, women working away from home is a large contributor to the decline of home cooking. (I'll take the trade-off, any day.)

Home cooking appears quite different from a century ago, as the rise of food processing (Chapter 4) and supermarkets that provide quick-scratch assists—whether from powdered sauces, canned soup, or cake mixes—has redefined the act. (And even serious home cooks regularly turn to ingredients like packaged butter and bouillon and jarred condiments for ease.) Three out of four participating in the above Harris Poll reported using pre-prepped or frozen foods to assist with cooking, for example. Plus, Americans report that they simply have less time in general, and cooking is not a high priority for most in these early decades of the 21st century—nor is it a necessity. These shifts in lifestyle and values have created the space for novel foodstuffs and new markets. Products like Rice-a-Roni, Hamburger Helper, and Kraft Macaroni & Cheese have been around for decades to help busy people cook. But the new millennium has seen an escalating number of fancier products grace supermarket shelves, further limiting the time and steps individuals need to get a hot meal on the table.

The inevitable development of this trend, of course, is that supermarkets now sell foods that require no added ingredients. Most reading this will think first—and probably fondly—of their favorite spot for rotisserie chicken: Supper is served! While those tasty birds still dominate sales in grocery delis, supermarkets today offer a buffet (literally) of fully prepared hot meals. Another study showed that, over one month, 58% of seniors and 78% of millennials purchased fresh prepared foods, which hit the sweet spot for "time-starved, quality-seeking consumers between choices of costlier restaurant meals and less-catchy, more laborious packaged goods," according to "Supermarket Guru" Phil Lempert.

Another new variant in the "cook at home" category is meal kits, in which boxes are delivered to doorsteps and include both ingredients and recipes. The kits take much of the time and effort out of preparing a meal, and the concept has taken off in kitchens in the US and England in recent years. Though meal kits may seem poised to take over home cooking, an NPD 2016 survey estimates that this "niche" market only included about 3% (8 million) of American adults. Though more than 150 companies compete for this $1.5 billion market, it's less than 1% of total food sales. That said, NPD found that about 20% (50 million) of consumers are interested in trying meal kits, suggesting the trend will continue growing and diversifying. In the UK, for example, Weight Watchers jumped into the game in 2017 as another option to reach overweight consumers.

How meals are consumed has also changed. Today, a greater percentage of American adults eat alone, reflecting smaller households and differing priorities. In the US, for example, Census Bureau data indicate that 27% of households contained a single person in 2012, up from 17% in 1970; the number is now about 33%, as in other places, like Korea. Data from roughly the same time period reflected a three-fold increase in the percentage of Americans dining alone, whether at a restaurant, at their car or desk, or in the home. The NPD Group found that breakfast was the meal most commonly consumed alone (60%), followed by lunch (55%), then dinner (32%).

Dining alone can be more, or less, healthful depending on a variety of factors. Eating with others in social settings tends to lead to larger portions and less attention paid to internal satiety signals, for example, while noshing with health-conscious folks can have a positive impact. And whether eating alone "could actually kill you" seems quite unlikely, as several headlines sensationalized after one study found that eating two or more meals alone each day was associated with a higher risk of T2DM and CVD (cardiovascular disease). Many other factors come into play that were not considered by the study, like what was eaten, in what circumstances, and other lifestyle factors.

One group for whom eating together is important, however, is kids; and the role of family meals in children's health has received considerable research attention. A meta-analysis of 17 studies of kids aged 2–17 years found that those consuming 3 or more family meals per week were 24% more likely to eat nutritious foods and

12% less likely to be overweight, eat unhealthy foods (20%), or have disordered eating (35%). Conversely, eating in front of the television or other screens has been associated with poorer eating habits and overweight in a number of studies, especially among children. A 2017 review of 13 studies found that watching television was associated with higher intakes of sugary foods and beverages and lower intakes of fruit and vegetables, though few of them considered factors that may confound the association.

The frequency of family dinners has decreased during the past century, as well as in recent decades, a change related to more women working and busier-than-ever kids. And so has the meaning of "family dinner," with some percentage of meals happening in front of the television or in the presence of electronic devices like smart phones. Still, families dine together more often than is generally assumed: Gallup reported that 5.1 dinners per week were eaten on average as a family in 2013, down slightly from 5.4 in 1997. And the same 2014 NPD survey found that about half of all families surveyed ate dinner with their kids at least 5 times per week.

Does snacking or meal timing matter?

Whether at home or not, a big change in eating behavior has been the movement from three main meals to snacking, or grazing, throughout the day. Snacking has been on the rise since the 1970s and comprises an increasingly larger part of Americans' daily energy intake across all ages. And the sheer diversity of snacks has conflated the definition of a meal. In 2015, 45% of meals included snack foods, for example. And snacks on their own, especially those from fast food drive-in windows, make for quick consumption right from the driver's seat: the 2005 Dashboard Dining study polled a random sample of those leaving a drive-through and found that 30% ate in their car at least twice weekly. (Taco Bell's Crunchwrap Supreme ranked most convenient, in case you were wondering.)

Research on whether smaller meals throughout the day or larger meals consumed less frequently are better for health is ongoing. For those whose blood sugar is less stable, eating smaller meals more frequently can be helpful, while for others snacking throughout the day simply adds excess calories. Conversely, there are physiological

benefits to resting your body from constant consumption and digestion, as in intermittent fasting (Chapter 17). And some snacks are
clearly better than others—just as some meals are better than others.
Timing may yet end up being important due to factors like circadian rhythms. A few recent studies suggest that front-loading
calories—eating the biggest meal at breakfast with a subsequently
smaller lunch and dinner—is associated with lower weight and
better biomarkers due to differences in hunger and satiety hormones
that shift throughout the day and night. Insulin, for example, is more
active in the morning compared to nighttime, facilitating energy metabolism that favors higher calorie intake earlier in the day. Indeed,
one study showed more than twice the weight loss among women
eating their largest meal at breakfast compared to those eating it at
dinnertime—despite consuming a similar number of calories and
foods. Still, evidence is far from conclusive, and larger studies and
randomized controlled trials are needed to establish cause and effect.
For now, focusing on the "what" and "how much," not the "when,"
appears most important. Consuming a nutritious diet that balances
calories is the key: one size doesn't fit all, and various combinations
of meals and snacks can work (Chapter 17).

How do restaurants, cafeterias, and other "away-from-home" options impact diet?

Supermarkets now compete with restaurants for food dollars due
to increased quality and quantity of prepared food offerings at com-
petitive prices that people bring to their own table. Yet eating away
from home continues to be a big part of how humans dine in today's
world, and the days are long gone when restaurants were just for
special occasions.

In the US, the percent of daily calories coming from outside the
home has risen during the past several decades, now at 28% in low-
income households and 31% and 35% in middle- and high-income
households, respectively. Said another way, 43% of household food
expenditures today were spent outside the home compared to 26% in
1970. These "away-from-home" numbers also include food eaten in
such places as school and workplace cafeterias, though restaurants
of all kinds are also in the mix, from formal dining to quick service

and fast food, with everything in between to meet every style and budget. Fast food in particular has shown major growth, from 6% of calories consumed in 1977 to 16% in 2012. Specifically, children consumed 14% of daily calories on average from fast food in 2012, up from 4% in 1977–78. Our proclivity for dining out is driving the industry: restaurant jobs in 2017 grew faster than healthcare, construction, or manufacturing in the US, 50% of which were in sit-down restaurants and 37% in fast food spots. They are expected to overtake manufacturing by 2020, another indicator of the expanding service economy.

Americans aren't the only ones for whom eating out is simply a way of life. The 2016 Nielsen Global Health and Ingredient-Sentiment Survey of Internet users in 63 countries found that 48% of people around the world eat at restaurants at least once weekly— and almost 1 in 10 (9%) do so at least daily. Those in North America (31%) and Asia-Pacific (28%) reported dining out once or twice a week most frequently, followed by those in Latin America (21%), Africa/Middle East (20%), and Europe (14%). Away-from-home options are often grouped into either quick-service (street food, fast food, cafeterias) or sit-down (casual dining, formal restaurant, café) locales. Of these, fast food and casual joints were the most popular dining choices by far, with food cost being the largest driver of where to eat, followed by food quality. Interestingly, only a very small percentage selected "not enough time to prepare my own meal" as a driver of dining out: 5% in North America and 7% in the other four regions.

Food outside the home can be as healthy as home-cooked meals, depending on one's cooking skills and nutrition knowledge. But the dearth of dietary information like ingredients and calorie counts on restaurant offerings, often the norm, does not help discerning consumers. At the same time, many restaurants encourage overconsumption, whether through complimentary bread, "supersizing," or tantalizing food that's just too tempting to turn down. And many studies have found that food outside the home tends to be higher in total calories, saturated fat, cholesterol, sodium, and refined carbohydrates and lower in nutrients like fiber and iron compared to home-cooked meals. A growing body of research also suggests that the increasing prevalence of dining out is a likely contributor to the growth of diet-related diseases in the US and globally.

Cafeterias in workplaces, schools, and institutions (e.g., hospitals) provide additional spaces for away-from-home eating. American kids today, for example, consume as much as 50% of their daily calories at school, and more than 31 million public school children are served annually by the National School Lunch Program (NSLP, est. 1946).[3] NSLP often comes under fire, as it and similar programs don't always reflect current nutrition science—especially when at odds with explicit aims to encourage consumption of agricultural commodities like milk and meat. Still, school programs, many of which now include breakfast, are critical in providing free meals for kids who might otherwise go hungry. And newer initiatives, like USDA's Farm to School Program (est. 2012), aim to increase overall food awareness through school gardens, nutrition education, and cooking classes.

As in schools, workplace cafeterias are fundamental components of the foodscape—and so, too, does nutritional quality vary. Efforts to improve offerings in both spaces include increasing the availability and decreasing the price of healthy foods, posting nutrition information, and offering cooking demonstrations. One workplace study, for instance, found that salad bar sales more than tripled when the cost was lowered—but returned to baseline levels when the price returned to normal. Other strategies, like the "traffic light" system labeling foods as red, yellow, or green to cue consumption, have also been effective, as has changing the placement of foods in the cafeteria ("choice architecture") to stimulate healthy purchases.

The increasing appreciation for wellbeing in productivity, in tandem with shifting values focused on not only nutritious but also sustainable food options—think fully recyclable or reusable utensils and plates, no plastic bottles or water coolers, a return to water fountains—is leading to ever more positive changes in food environments in schools, workplaces, hospitals, and other institutions that serve hundreds of millions around the world each day.

What roles do street food and food trucks play?

Tens of millions of people consume "street food" daily, defined by the Food and Agriculture Organization of the United Nations (FAO) as "ready-to-eat food and beverages prepared and/or sold by vendors or hawkers, especially in the street and other similar places." It is a major contributor of calories for some, especially low- and middle-income city dwellers in Asia, Latin America, and Africa. Street foods are easy to access, inexpensive, and provide income for those for whom employment may be otherwise unlikely, often women. In Bangkok, a 2012 FAO report estimated that 20 000+ vendors provided 40% of calorie intake for city dwellers between 2005 and 2011.

While there is much good (and deliciousness) that comes from street food, negative effects abound from the lack of infrastructure and regulations, including garbage and wastewater in the streets and traffic congestion. Human rights violations are also a concern in some places due to child labor. The largest concern with street food is foodborne illness (Chapter 2). As a result, FAO and others have been working with governments to help hawkers improve food safety handling. Increasing the healthfulness of street foods has been another priority because they tend to be tasty nibbles that aren't always the best choice nutritionally. Exceptions exist, though: a study in Calcutta found that a meal costing about 5 Indian rupees (less than 10 cents in US dollars) included 1000 calories, 30 g of protein, 15 g of fat, and 180 g of carbohydrates, comparable nutritionally to home meals.

The food truck is the newest addition[4] to the street food scene in higher-income countries, a trend that began in the US but recently hit London with its food tent "gazebos." The phenomenon exploded in the 21st century, spreading to urbanites around the country hungry for the next new thing in food. *Smithsonian* food writer Jonathan Gold attributes the spark to Roy Choi in 2008, whose successful Korean taco truck in Los Angeles, Kogi, began a movement. Today, more and more inspired cooks and entrepreneurs are turning to food trucks rather than traditional brick-and-mortar restaurants to bring their eats directly to people while keeping overhead low. Gold further muses that food trucks are not only deeply social experiences but also "a vehicle for traversing lines of race, class, and ethnicity."

And so they are—like so many other food encounters.

Part III

ESSENTIAL FOOD
AND NUTRITION

SEPARATING SCIENCE FROM
JUNK SCIENCE

While many subfields of nutrition science have emerged, the discipline is rooted in biochemistry. Its foundation is the mighty micronutrients and phytonutrients and the major energy sources—fat, carbohydrate, and protein—that make up our everyday diets. The knowledge of how what we eat impacts our bodies can then be used to inform health promotion and disease prevention programs and guidelines for individuals and communities alike, and applied to directly enhance the healthfulness of the food supply.

6

A BRIEF HISTORY OF NUTRITION

SCIENTIFIC DISCOVERIES AND APPLICATIONS

How do we know what we know about food and health?

We eat every day, and we know how food makes us feel. Perhaps because of this, many overlook that nutrition is a discipline dedicated to understanding how what we eat and drink impacts our health and risk of disease, a life science that grew out of analytical chemistry. The *Oxford English Dictionary* defines nutrition as "1. The process of providing or obtaining the food necessary for health and growth; 1.1. Food; nourishment; 1.2. The branch of science that deals with nutrients and nutrition, particularly in humans." The word "nutrient" refers to a chemical necessary for nourishment and growth. In nutrition, there are six essential classes of nutrients: fat, carbohydrate, and protein (together known as "macronutrients"); vitamins and minerals (together known as "micronutrients"); and water. Nutrients can be delivered in diverse packages, whether food or drink, pill or powder. However consumed, they are digested and metabolized and distribute nourishment throughout the body. Each of the nutrients discussed in this chapter (except water; Chapter 14) has unique physiochemical properties whose bioactivity impacts health, longevity, and wellbeing.

Humans have been observing how food impacts health over the course of human evolution. Hunter–gatherers learned, for example, that food led to either pleasure or pain, sustenance or death; and thus history progressed with tales passed from generation to generation. Skip (way) forward to classical Greece, where Hippocrates (c.400 BCE), the so-called Father of Western Medicine, is credited with the adage "Let thy food be thy medicine." Before then, ancient India gave birth to Ayurveda ("the science of life"), a system of medicine more concerned with mind–body connections than traditional Western practice. The Vedas (Sanskrit for "knowledge" or "wisdom") were first described as early as 5000 BCE; they are the oldest sacred texts, dated between the second and first millennia BCE, from which Ayurveda later developed into a systematic science with its roots in food and herbs as keys to good health and wellbeing. Around the same time, China was developing its own theories in a similar fashion, now referred to as traditional Chinese medicine.

Though Hippocrates' words are catchy—and apt—food is far more than medicine. Ayurveda and other holistic philosophies arguably possess a more sophisticated understanding of the power of food and the meaning of total health than traditional Western medicine. This is because Western practice and philosophy focus on treatment (ergo, "medicine") and have historically disregarded the power of prevention in general, and nutrition in particular. Happily, Eastern and Western philosophies continue to edge closer to each other as Eastern practices now receive public research dollars to test age-old hypotheses. In the meantime, much of what we know today about food and health arises from Western methodologies born during the Scientific Revolution and beyond.

How did the study of food become the science of nutrition?

The late Renaissance period in 16th-century Europe saw a resurging interest in observing and measuring the natural world through disciplines like physics, biology, chemistry, and mathematics, a time described as the "Scientific Revolution." "Father of Empiricism" Francis Bacon (1561–1626) wrote, "There remains simple experience; which, if taken as it comes, is called accident, if sought for, experiment. The true method of experience first lights the candle [hypothesis], and then by means of the candle shows the way [arranges and delimits the experiment]; commencing as it does with experience duly ordered and digested, not bungling or erratic, and from it deducing axioms [theories], and from established axioms again new experiment." Bacon's tenets are the basis of the scientific method: stating a general research problem and question, articulating a specific study question to examine the phenomenon, stating a hypothesis, testing the hypothesis by collecting data systematically, interpreting data, and formulating conclusions. The final step is to conduct additional experiments to replicate the findings and reformulate the hypothesis as needed. Theories eventually emerge to explain a group of related phenomena. Still today, the use of the scientific method remains the sole criterion that differentiates science from anecdote, fact from opinion.

Yet it wasn't until the "Chemical Revolution" in France during the late 18th century that food and health became the subject of systematic scientific inquiry. Employing the tools of analytical chemistry allowed scientists to begin answering fundamental questions like "How is food metabolized?" In 1770, "Father of Nutrition and Chemistry" Antoine Lavoisier demonstrated that food reacted with oxygen in the body to release heat and water. Later studies in the 1800s investigated the chemical composition of food itself, finding that all victuals included carbon, hydrogen, and oxygen, while some also contained nitrogen. Nitrogen's unique role in health and longevity stimulated research in both animal models and plant crops. "Protein" (1839) was among the first major discoveries in the still-nascent nutrition science and the focus of numerous studies and feeding trials.

During these decades, many scientists explored the basic chemistry of macronutrient (fat, carbohydrate, protein) composition, metabolism, and digestion. Others focused on diseases hypothesized to have a nutritional cause, based on observations of populations who shared a common diet. Diseases related to micronutrient deficiencies were rampant, and during the next century research would lead to the discovery of vitamins and minerals and, later, the synthesis of some of these chemicals for addition to the food supply. Iodine-rich salt, for example, was found to prevent goiter through its role in thyroid functioning (1850). Polished white rice lacked vitamin B_1 and therefore caused beriberi (1897).

A noteworthy example of a study addressing nutrient deficiency was conducted by James Lind, a British physician. Lind saw that British sailors were dying during long sea voyages, observations that had also been made around 200 years prior. In what is thought to be the first ever intervention study, or clinical trial, Lind provided lemons and oranges to some sailors as part of their diet but not others (the control group), learning that the group receiving citrus did not develop the disease. Additional research later showed that some leafy greens and other citrus fruits also prevented scurvy. But it wasn't until the 1940s, more than 400 years after the first observations of scurvy, and about 175 years following Lind's trial, that vitamin C (ascorbic acid) was identified as the root cause.

Nutrition scientists today still show compelling associations between food and disease without knowing the bioactive component responsible for the effect. Lind's trial, and countless other examples, underscores the importance of food-based research in nutrition science: we don't always fully understand why something is happening that leads to reduced disease and suffering (i.e., the mechanism), but the science will eventually catch up. Even so, as nutrition science progressed the discipline became dominated by reductionist studies focused on nutrients, rather than foods. Though single-nutrient studies can be illustrative, they can also lead scientists astray when other salient dietary components are not considered in concert, or in the context of an overall diet (Chapter 17).

What is nutrification? What is fortification?

While guidelines and recommendations, policies and programs, are all important, the most powerful application of nutrition knowledge to improve health, arguably, is to add nutrients directly to foods. "Nutrification" refers to the process of increasing the nutrient content of a food to improve the dietary intake of a population. Scientist Paul Bauernfeind calls it "the most rapidly applied, most flexible, and most socially acceptable form of public health intervention designed to improve the health of a population without requiring education or behavior modification."

A common method of nutrifying foods is fortification, defined by the Food and Agriculture Organization (FAO) and the World Health Organization (WHO) as "deliberately increasing the content of essential micronutrients in a food so as to improve the nutritional quality of the food supply and provide a public health benefit with minimal risk to health." Fortification programs may be mandated by law or initiated voluntarily by industry. Foods are selected for nutrient delivery based on the degree to which a population regularly consumes them, a region-specific assessment. (Alternatives exist: vitamin supplements in the form of powders or pills can be delivered directly to individuals or households, for instance, if food fortification isn't feasible.) The three major fortification programs employed globally provide vitamin A, iron, and iodine, all of which reduce pain and suffering and mortality, decrease healthcare costs, and curtail lost economic productivity and income.

Iodine, for example, is required for proper functioning of the thyroid gland, and inadequate intakes result in a large neck growth (goiter). Low iodine during pregnancy and early childhood seriously compromises neurological development, leading to severe intellectual disability. Early Chinese writings (c.3600 BCE) recorded decreases in goiter following consumption of sea vegetables, and research in the early 19th century identified iodine as the responsible nutrient. Endemic iodine deficiency was observed around the world as well as in the US "goiter belt" (Great Lakes, Appalachia, Northwest) in the early 20th century. Iodized salt was first sold in Michigan in 1924, following a successful program in Switzerland. Today, more than 120 countries mandate salt fortification. It remains voluntary in the US, though; thus, the American Thyroid Association and the Endocrine Society recommend that women take an iodine supplement during preconception for optimal fetal development (depending on their diet and where they live).

Fortification programs have evolved alongside nutrition knowledge, and more recent applications include the prevention of chronic diseases and birth defects. For instance, an association between folate deficiency and neural tube defects (NTDs) was first hypothesized in 1965. Randomized controlled trials (RCTs) in England and Hungary initially showed that supplementation during early pregnancy was protective. Research evidence accumulated, and the early 1990s saw increased efforts in the US to educate women of childbearing age to consume a folate supplement, as the effects occur during the first 28 days of conception, often before a woman is aware of the pregnancy. Experts eventually suggested folate fortification as a better means to prevent NTDs. The US, Canada, and Costa Rica first implemented mandatory fortification in 1998, followed by

Chile (2000) and South Africa (2003). Grain-containing foods like breakfast cereals and bread were nutrified with folate in the US. Subsequent studies showed a 19–32% decrease in NTDs such as spina bifida and anencephaly, leading some to call folic acid fortification "one of the most successful public health initiatives in the past 50–75 years." Still, there are always potential adverse consequences from fortification programs, and some have considered whether the increased consumption of folate among those *not* at risk for NTDs may lead to an increased risk of heart disease and some cancers. While studies have not shown deleterious impacts thus far, research is ongoing.

The addition of the prefix "bio" to the word "fortification" refers to nutrification through conventional plant breeding and agronomic practices (e.g., selecting cereals for high protein or iron content) or through genetic modification (e.g., modifying genes to produce nutrients). The goal of biofortification is to increase nutritional content during production rather than processing "to reach populations where supplementation and conventional fortification activities may be difficult to implement and/or limited," according to WHO. Current biofortification projects around the world include beta-carotene (vitamin A) in sweet potato, maize, and cassava; zinc in wheat, rice, beans, maize, and sweet potato; iron in rice, beans, legumes, cassava, and sweet potato; and protein and amino acids in sorghum and cassava. "Golden rice" is another example, in which genetic engineering is used to create a rice that produces beta-carotene to combat vitamin A deficiency (VAD; Chapter 2). The project began in 1982 and the first strain was successfully created in 1999. Many studies have since shown that golden rice can help mitigate VAD. Unfortunately, the crop has struggled due to violent anti-science sentiment and activity, including a 2013 incident when activists destroyed farms undergoing field trials, setting back its progress greatly. There is some indication that genetically engineered (GE) rice may come to market in the near future.

Fortification programs are indeed among public health's greatest success stories and continue saving countless lives each year all around the world where they are employed—and result in tragic, completely preventable deaths where they are not.

What other methods are used to nutrify foods?

Enrichment, restoration, and supplementation are additional methods that alter nutrient composition. "Enriched" is sometimes used synonymously with "fortified," although in the US it is a legal term that means a food must contain 10% or more of the daily nutrient value compared to the same nonenriched food. Restoration involves adding back nutrients originally present before food processing; adding vitamins and minerals back to refined white flour (Chapter 10) is a familiar example. "Supplementation" refers to any product designed to enhance nutritional intake and can take the familiar form of a pill (e.g., vitamin, mineral, herb, amino acid) or any other delivery vehicle (e.g., liquid extract, powder). Supplements can be lifesavers, whether as infant formulas in places where breastfeeding is not possible or as complete nutritional shakes for those suffering from health conditions impacting appetite. Conversely, some dietary supplements are expensive products with excessive (non)nutrients that might either lack a solid research base or employ an ineffective chemical formulation. In the worst-case scenario, supplements may be adulterated or contaminated, creating a serious health risk. (The dietary supplement industry is an important topic beyond the scope of this book; those taking supplements should conduct due diligence on the purity and dose of the product and consult with a nutrition professional.)

While adding essential nutrients to foods to save lives still happens through nutrification efforts like fortification, today's clever industrialists create copious multivitamin, multimineral products with (perceived) added value, from vitamin-enhanced waters to protein power bars and everything in between. Products like these are often referred to as "nutraceuticals" or "functional foods," late-20th-century terms that describe the act of making food more nutritious to meet (or create) a consumer desire. Yet other products load vitamins and minerals into foods without paying much attention to fundamentals like macronutrient composition, ingredients, and calorie content. A Coca-Cola variant with added fiber comes to mind, as do 100% whole grain breakfast cereals loaded in sugar. There are thousands of these types of foods, and it's not always clear that they "improve" diets; nutrition knowledge (and common sense) is needed to facilitate informed choices. Thus, while many of today's products are departures from the original intent of nutrification—to directly prevent or manage disease and save lives—applications will continue to evolve, providing ever more options for consumers to create diets that meet diverse needs and lifestyles.

7

SMALL AND MIGHTY

VITAMINS, MINERALS, AND PHYTONUTRIENTS

What are vitamins?

Vitamins are organic compounds (i.e., contain carbon) essential for life that must be obtained in the diet because they cannot be synthesized by the body. They are generally classified as water- or fat-soluble and often appear on ingredient lists with either their common or chemical names.

- **Fat-soluble vitamins**: A (retinol, retinal, retinoic acid), D (calciferol, cholecalciferol), E (tocopherol), and K (phylloquinone, menoquinone)
- **Water-soluble vitamins**: B_1 (thiamin), B_2 (riboflavin), B_3 (niacin, nicotinic acid), B_5 (pantothenic acid), B_6 (pyridoxal, pyridoxine, pyridoxamine), B_{12} (cobalamin), C (ascorbic acid, ascorbate), folate (folic acid, folacin), biotin, and choline

Vitamins have various chemical forms that impact biological function—there are alpha- and gamma-tocopherols, for example. They play multifarious roles throughout the body, including in eye health and immune function (vitamin A), bone and dental health (vitamin D), blood clotting (vitamin K), and prevention of diseases like spina bifida and heart disease (folate). The B vitamins act as cofactors in metabolic processes that convert food into energy, and newer research focuses on their roles in cognitive functioning and isease, among others. (A free vitamin fact sheet is available wby.com.)

The ability to dissolve in water impacts how vitamins are metabolized. Water-soluble vitamins are easily absorbed in our aqueous bodies, and, while tiny amounts are stored temporarily, excesses are excreted in urine. Fat-soluble vitamins are, as their name implies, best absorbed in the presence of fat. (It's this principle of nutritional biochemistry that explains why you'll want to keep that yummy full-fat vinaigrette on your salad: the oils in the dressing will help your body absorb the fat-soluble vitamins from your vegetables.) Fat-soluble vitamins can build up in our adipose tissue (body fat). In rare cases, such as people with extremely high vitamin supplement intakes, levels of fat-soluble vitamins can become toxic and even fatal.

Billions globally suffer from severe vitamin deficiencies (Chapter 2), but, with some exceptions, most of those living in food-abundant areas have intakes that prevent frank deficiencies—particularly due to food fortification efforts. Whether consumption of specific vitamins is adequate for "optimal" health, athletic performance, cognition, or disease prevention, is a more difficult question to answer, and research is ongoing.

What's the deal with vitamin D?

Those who follow nutrition news may have noticed vitamin D is the "it" vitamin. It is found in limited food sources naturally (like fatty fish), so milk and other foods are fortified in many places to prevent deficiencies like rickets, a bone disease. The "sunshine vitamin" is primarily synthesized in the skin when ultraviolet B rays (UVB) react with the hormone 7-dehydrocholesterol; humans with darker skin have more melanin, which impedes vitamin D production. Research has demonstrated that humans in northern climes have significantly lower concentrations of vitamin D in their blood compared to southern-clime dwellers. Concentrations also vary within region due to lifestyle differences (e.g., use of sunscreen, time outdoors) that compromise sunlight exposure.

Vitamin D plays diverse roles in the body, in part by regulating calcium and phosphorus, both of which play a key role in bone and dental health. Yet newer hypotheses regarding the role of vitamin D in chronic diseases like cancer, obesity, and type 2 diabetes mellitus (T2DM) suggest that lower blood concentrations may lead to higher risks, though research is not conclusive. While some scientists claim an epidemic of vitamin D deficiency may be contributing to the burden of chronic disease, there is not yet a clear consensus on optimal blood concentrations of vitamin D, though many experts believe that individuals should delay sunscreen application to enable vitamin D production or take high-dose supplements. More will be discovered about vitamin D in coming years pending completion of ongoing clinical trials.

How do you know whether your vitamin intake is adequate? Should you take a supplement?

In food-abundant environments, micronutrient needs are often met by consuming a balanced and varied diet (Chapter 17). Nonetheless, a 2015 report from the US Department of Agriculture (USDA) indicates a number of micronutrient imbalances among Americans: vitamin A, vitamin D, vitamin E, folate, vitamin C, calcium, magnesium, potassium, and fiber were underconsumed across all groups; sodium was overconsumed; and iron was underconsumed by adolescent, premenopausal, and pregnant females. Other data suggest that vitamins B_6 and B_{12} were low in older adults. With so many micronutrients to consider in so many different circumstances, isn't it easier to take a multivitamin or mineral supplement as part of your daily routine?

While intuitively appealing—and a source of billions for the supplement industry—studies showing consistently positive health benefits of daily multivitamin/multimineral consumption have been disappointing. This is likely due to many factors: those taking supplements are often already generally healthy; supplement quality varies widely in the market; and chemical forms differ in their absorption and bioactivity, hence efficacy. For example, over-the-counter supplements may be synthesized at dangerously high doses or at ineffectively low doses or adulterated with inert or toxic chemicals due to the insufficient regulatory environment in some countries—including the US, where the 1994 Dietary Supplement Health and Education Act (DSHEA) allows manufacturers to circumvent the lengthy scrutiny and approval process required by other drugs. While many consider a supplement a form of "dietary insurance," it's best to aim to meet your micronutrient needs from food, which tend to carry fewer risks and greater benefits. Specific clinical, age-related, or other needs requiring supplementation should be considered in conjunction with a nutrition professional as part of an overall health strategy.

What roles do salt and other minerals play in our diet, and should you watch your sodium intake? What is the DASH diet?

Minerals are inorganic substances that enter our food supply, hence our bodies, through the soil in which plants grow (or via animals that eat the plants). The mineral content of the same crop can therefore differ somewhat by geography and climate. There are seven macrominerals (calcium, chloride, sodium, potassium, phosphorus, magnesium, sulfur) and nine trace minerals (aka, microminerals: chromium, copper, fluoride, iodine, iron, manganese, molybdenum, selenium, and zinc), so named because of the quantities needed for health.

Like vitamins, minerals play an array of roles in the body. For example, chromium and glucose support metabolism; magnesium, sodium, and potassium regulate blood pressure; and fluoride improves dental health. Life-threatening mineral deficiencies are rare in high-income countries but serious health problems occur from them in low- and middle-income countries (Chapter 2). As with vitamin research, many mineral studies today focus not just on deficiencies but on roles in chronic disease prevention as well as athletic performance. Knowledge in these areas will continue to grow. (A free mineral fact sheet is available at pknewby.com.)

Sodium plays a vital role in fluid balance, which regulates blood pressure, as well as in muscle contractions and nerve impulses. While most people use the word "sodium" interchangeably with "salt," sodium is actually only one component of table salt, which is a combination of sodium and chloride. (There are other salts, for example, like potassium chloride.) Research is convincing that high intakes of sodium increase blood pressure and hypertension, risk factors for heart disease and stroke. Modest salt reduction for at least four weeks leads to reduced blood pressure, as shown in a systematic review and meta-analysis of 34 RCTs and many individual studies. People vary in their sensitivity to salt, however, which explains why sodium intake doesn't always correlate with blood pressure; hypertension has strong genetic components independent of diet, and obesity is also a major risk factor. Monitoring blood pressure regularly is critical: hypertension is a "silent killer" that can be controlled with medication if unresponsive to diet and other lifestyle changes. For these reasons, individuals should limit their sodium intake to less than 5000 mg per day according to the World Health Organization (WHO) (<2300 mg is the US recommendation). A sprinkle or two of salt in cooking or at the table is not the culprit, however; cutting back on high-sodium processed foods (Chapter 4) is the key.

Because sodium does not act alone in regulating blood pressure, studies have also examined the roles of minerals like magnesium, potassium, and calcium, suggesting that the ratio is key to blood pressure control, not just sodium. The overall diet is also important. The Dietary Approaches to Stop Hypertension (DASH) research team has been examining the role of nutrition in blood pressure reduction for decades through a series of RCTs comparing those consuming a typical Western-style (American) diet with those who either just increased fruits and vegetables or followed the DASH diet. The DASH eating plan includes an array of plant-based foods (vegetables, fruits, whole grains, beans, legumes) plus low-fat dairy, lean protein, and vegetable oils and limits saturated fat and foods high in sugar. Those adding fruits and vegetables to a typical American diet showed reductions in blood pressure as well as low-density lipoprotein ("bad") cholesterol (LDL) compared to those consuming a typical American diet, but those following the DASH diet showed the greatest reductions. The DASH diet combined with reduced sodium (3000 versus 2300 or 1500 mg/day) showed increasingly greater blood pressure reduction with the lower sodium intakes. The DASH diet has also been shown to be effective for weight loss (Chapter 17). Beyond the original DASH RCTs, numerous observational studies, meta-analyses, and systematic reviews have found a consistently protective effect of the DASH diet on blood pressure and other cardiovascular risk factors, as well as heart disease and stroke.

What are phytochemicals?

Phytochemicals are organic compounds (i.e., contain carbon) found across the plant kingdom—*phyto* refers to plants in Greek—including fruits, vegetables, whole grains, nuts, tea, cocoa, and coffee. The words "phytochemical" and "phytonutrient" are used interchangeably in nutrition. Approximately 100 000 phytochemicals have been characterized, and doubtless many more will be discovered. Phytochemicals provide protection for plants, whether as brightly colored pigments that fight predators or as colorless chemicals that act as antioxidants to boost immunity. It's little wonder they have beneficial effects in humans given their importance in plant health: "You are what you eat," as the saying goes. Because there are so many, phytonutrients are often categorized by chemical structure or biological activity. Four major groups are discussed below.

Carotenoids are usually red, orange, yellow, or green and include a number of different chemicals that can be converted into vitamin A in the body ("pro-vitamin A" beta-carotene, alpha-carotene, beta-cryptoxanthin) and those that cannot (lycopene, lutein, zeaxanthin). Some studies have shown associations between carotenoids and decreased heart disease and certain cancers, likely due to their antioxidant activity. Lycopene (found in tomatoes, especially when cooked) is related to lower risk of prostate cancer, and beta-carotene (found in carrots and other orange and yellow veggies) may be associated with decreased lung cancer in nonsmokers. Lutein and zeaxanthin seem to protect against age-related macular degeneration and cataracts, serious eye diseases that compromise sight in older adults. Carotenoids are fat-soluble and must be consumed with fat in order to be absorbed; excess carotenoids are stored in the subcutaneous fat under the skin, so if you munch carrots excessively, your skin may take on an orange hue. (Seriously.)

Polyphenols are the largest group of phytochemicals across the food supply, and include flavonoids and nonflavonoids (referring to the chemical structure). Bioactive roles in the body differ, but most impact nutrient metabolism and absorption. Some current polyphenol research efforts include catechins in tea; quercetin in onions; flavonones in citrus; resveratrol, a flavonol, in red grape skins, wine, and peanuts; anthocyanins in apples; and ellagic acid in berries and pomegranates. High intakes of a wide range of colorful polyphenols may promote longevity due to antioxidant and anti-inflammatory effects.

Phytoestrogens are named because of their estrogen-like effects on the body, though some have additional health impacts. They are colorless or white, and major types include isoflavones and lignans, found in tofu and other soy foods and flax and sesame seeds, respectively (Chapter 11). Decades of research has investigated their association with hormone-related processes like the development of breast cancer and osteoporosis. Results on the role of isoflavones in reproductive cancers have been mixed, although foods rich in phytoestrogens have long been part of the traditional diet in Okinawa, Japan, whose inhabitants are among the longest-lived populations in the world (Chapter 17).

Glucosinolates are sulfur-containing compounds responsible for the bitter and spicy flavors of some cruciferous vegetables (e.g., kale, broccoli, Brussels sprouts, cabbage, cauliflower, turnip, radish) and leafy greens (e.g., collards, mustard, horseradish, wasabi, arugula). They are metabolized into isothiocyanates and indoles, which have been related to a lower risk of colorectal and other cancers due to their role in hormone metabolism, among other functions. Although rare, high doses of glucosinolates can disturb thyroid function; adequate iodine intake generally prevents ill outcomes, though, and most people should consume more glucosinolate-rich foods, not fewer.

Do carotenoids prevent cancer?

Carotenoids have received considerable attention in laboratory and animal models, later leading to observational studies in humans and then clinical trials. (This is a natural progression of etiologic research necessary for establishing cause and effect.) It was hypothesized in the 1990s that high-dose supplementation may prevent lung cancer given the protective role of carotenoid-rich vegetables and fruits. Contrary to hypothesized, carotenoids provided in RCTs actually led to more deaths. The interpretation of findings is complicated as the studies were conducted among those at high risk of lung cancer, like smokers (who may have had preclinical disease, for instance) and the dose was incredibly high. Still, some concluded that studies like these following a reductionist approach (i.e., picking out individual dietary elements from their complex, multinutrient food packages) are inherently limited given the many different bioactive and synergistic components in food. In other words, studies showing a health benefit of consuming carotenoid-rich foods like vegetables and fruits don't always neatly extrapolate to a protective effect based on high doses of just one of their phytochemicals, like beta-carotene. There may be other phytochemicals, nutrients, or as yet to be discovered components in veggies and fruits responsible for the cancer-reducing effect. Studies like these laid the groundwork for a paradigm shift in nutrition, with some scientists calling for a more holistic view of diet that better reflects the biochemical complexity of food—not to mention how people actually eat (i.e., meals, not nutrients) (Chapter 17).

8

THE FOUNDATION OF NUTRITION

CARBOHYDRATE, FAT, AND PROTEIN

What are the different kinds of carbohydrates we eat?

Carbohydrates are so named because of their chemical composition, which includes carbon, hydrogen, and oxygen. Globally, the main dietary carbohydrates are cereals, root and sugar crops, pulses (legumes), vegetables, fruit, and dairy. Each gram of carbohydrate provides about 4 calories, and "carbs" are the preferred energy source to fuel the brain and physical activity. Some carbohydrate is stored as glycogen, which constitutes approximately 10% of the liver's weight (~100 g) and 2% of muscle (~500 g). Liver glycogen maintains blood glucose (say, when sleeping), which requires tight regulation for proper body functioning. Muscle glycogen is the main source of energy during intensive exercise. Endurance athletes engage in "carb loading" to maximize muscle glycogen before a race and provide additional carbohydrates to the body for sustained physical activity.

Carbs are either digestible or indigestible and are considered monosaccharides, disaccharides, or polysaccharides; the prefix refers to the number of glucose units. Oligosaccharides (e.g., maltodextrin) are an additional class of carbs including 3–9 units. There are three monosaccharides in the diet: fructose (found in honey); galactose (found in milk); and glucose, also known as dextrose (found in table sugar). All digestible carbs are ultimately broken down into glucose. Blood glucose must be stable at all times and is tightly controlled through the hormone insulin, which moves glucose from the blood into cells for energy or storage. (Glucagon, insulin's opposite, releases glucose when blood sugar is low). Glucose dysregulation, often a result of malfunctioning of insulin and its receptors due to genetics and other factors, can result in either type 1 or type 2 diabetes mellitus (T2DM).

The monosaccharides glucose and galactose are quickly absorbed into the bloodstream, especially when consumed in liquid form, whereas fructose goes directly to the liver, where it's rapidly converted to glucose, glycogen, lactate, and fat. Disaccharides (i.e., double sugars) have two monosaccharides, and the three major ones in human diets are sucrose (glucose-fructose, found in table sugar, beet sugar, cane sugar), maltose (glucose-glucose, found in beer), and lactose (glucose-galactose, found in milk). Collectively, mono- and disaccharides are often referred to as "simple sugars" in nutrition, or just "sugars."

Polysaccharides are generally referred to as either starch or nonstarch (or fiber) and have at least 10 glucose units joined together, and often hundreds. Starch is the storage form of glucose found in plants and is particularly high in potatoes, corn, and wheat. Starches are sometimes referred to as "complex carbohydrates" because they have many more glucose units than simple sugars. Even so, they take a much shorter time to digest into glucose than you might expect. Research has shown that a high-starch, complex carb food like white bread has the same impact on blood glucose as table sugar, perhaps surprising to most eaters, as it lacks the fiber and other nutrients that help slow down digestion and absorption. And, in general, slowing digestion and absorption is a good thing for the body. Yet not all high-starch, complex carb foods are quickly digested and lead to spikes in blood sugar: it depends on the kind of starch. (It gets complicated, I know.) For instance, one form of starch, called "resistant starch" (RS), is found in plant foods like beans and legumes, especially lentils. Because RS is "resistant" to digestive enzymes, like fiber, it slows digestion and mitigates spikes in blood sugar, especially when consumed alongside other foods, as part of a meal. (Makes sense, right?)

Because of these varied impacts on blood sugar and blood insulin—hence risk of diseases like T2DM—some nutritionists employ a concept known as the "glycemic index" (GI) when thinking about the different types of carbs in the diet. High-carbohydrate diets filled with high-GI foods (e.g., sugary cakes, cookies, soda, white bread, white pasta) can create a large "glycemic load" (GL), a product of a food's GI in combination with its total carb content. Some studies show that individuals consuming a diet with a high GL have an increased risk for T2DM and heart disease. Even so, whether foods with a high GI are served hot or cold, how much they are cooked, and other physiochemical properties impact their effects in the body. Particularly important are the other foods they are consumed alongside: the nutrient composition of the whole meal matters.

What is fiber, and how is it related to health?

Fiber is sometimes referred to as "nondigestible carbohydrates" or "nonstarch polysaccharides." It comes mainly from the cell walls of plants and includes cellulose, hemicellulose, and pectin, though there are myriad fibers consumed by humans, not all of which are carbohydrates chemically (e.g., lignin). This is because "fiber" often refers to the physiological functions in the body and not just chemical composition. Most people consume inadequate fiber for health, less than half of the daily recommendation, which is around 25 g for women and 38 g for men in the US and 30 g daily for both in England.

Fiber is described as "insoluble" or "soluble." These terms refer to the ability to dissolve in water and undergo acid hydrolysis. Insoluble fibers are found mainly in cereal grains like wheat and corn bran as well as fruit skins. Fruit flesh (especially apples and citrus), beans, peas, oats, and barley are rich in soluble fiber; psyllium and beta-glucans have received a lot of research attention and may be particularly beneficial. Soluble fibers are more viscous and better fermented; they decrease the rate of glucose and lipid (fat) digestion and absorption, increase satiety, and lower LDL, a risk factor for heart disease. Insoluble fibers are slowly and incompletely fermented in the colon, producing fecal bulk and gas, a boon for colon health. There is a lot of overlap between the effects of soluble and insoluble fibers, however, and remembering which is which isn't important for everyday eaters who just want a sandwich. Moreover, resistant starches and some oligosaccharides (like inulin, found in artichokes) act like fibers even though they are not chemically nonstarch polysaccharides. This is why the Food and Agriculture Organization of the United Nations (FAO) recommends disregarding the soluble/insoluble nomenclature, and the Nutrition

Facts panel in the US reads simply "dietary fiber." What counts toward total dietary fiber intake will continue to evolve.

Hippocrates, known as the "Father of Modern Medicine," noted the beneficial effects of coarse wheat compared to refined wheat on laxation in 430 BCE. In the past century, fiber has received considerable research attention regarding its putative role in a wide array of health conditions and diseases because of its unique physiological and metabolic properties. In addition to its impacts on gut and bowel health, fiber is associated with lower body weight and a decreased risk of cardiovascular disease (CVD); links with cancers and T2DM are suggestive but remain equivocal. Cereal fibers, like wheat bran, are especially beneficial for stool bulk and healthy bowel habits. Oligosaccharides and resistant starch are known as "prebiotics." Prebiotics—found in such foods as leeks, artichokes, asparagus, garlic, oats, onions, soybeans, and wheat—are fermented in the gut to short-chain fatty acids, which provide energy to the colon (around 1–2 calories/g). They thus stimulate beneficial bacteria, resulting in healthier gut microflora (Chapter 4). Because fibers vary in their bioactivity, individuals should consume a variety rather than fixate on just one type. Fiber can impact absorption of minerals in theory, though the loss is not concerning for the vast majority; discuss your situation with a physician, particularly if you are taking a high-dose fiber supplement.

Are you eating the best carbs for your body? How do digestible carbohydrates, sugar, and high-fructose corn syrup differ?

Although digestible carbohydrates provide quick energy, most of us consume too many for optimal health. Digestible carbohydrates, particularly in the form of refined foods that lack fiber and other nutrients (like white bread and white pasta), are quickly metabolized to glucose and increase blood triglycerides (TGs), a type of fat stored in adipose (fat) tissue. High blood TGs are a risk factor for heart disease and T2DM, as well as fatty liver. Carbohydrates exceeding energy needs are also converted into fatty acids and then repackaged as TGs, leading to overweight and obesity. Whether carbs are used for energy or stored as fat depends on various things, including type and form of carbohydrate and genetics. Total body fat also matters, as adipose tissue is an active organ involved in myriad metabolic activities through its role in gene regulation and expression; biological parameters like free fatty acid concentration in the blood and insulin sensitivity also matter. Differences like these inform why high-carb diets evoke varied effects in different people, which may contribute one day to personalized nutrition (Chapter 18). Eaters can better understand whether their carb intake is healthful or harmful through regular checkups with a physician who measures a broad array of biomarkers, like blood glucose, blood insulin, blood TGs, and others.

Western diets are particularly abundant in simple sugars, a form of digestible carb that is often added to processed foods and stimulates our sweet tooth. These sugars are thus referred to as "added sugars" (to differentiate them from those found naturally in foods like fruit). Beet root, corn, sugar cane, and maple syrup are the major sources in the diet, though sugar has many guises when listed on ingredient lists: fruit juice concentrate, dextrose, invert sugar, malt syrup, anything with the word "cane" (like evaporated cane juice), and agave nectar are common. And "raw" or "natural" sugar is not superior to refined sugar; the touted nutritional differences are insignificant.

One simple sugar that receives tremendous attention is high-fructose corn syrup (HFCS). HFCS begins with corn sugar, to which fructose is added to enhance sweetness. It's a very common food ingredient for reasons including its liquid form and inexpensive price relative to other sugars. Given its ubiquity in the diet, many studies have examined whether HFCS and fructose might play a role in obesity and other chronic diseases. For instance, a 2016 systematic review and other studies have led a majority of scientists to conclude that HFCS does not play a specific role in obesity different from sucrose. This makes sense given the chemistry: Rippe and Angeloupoulos remind us that HFCS is comparable to sucrose, a disaccharide that also includes glucose and fructose, as each contains about the same amount of fructose, or about 50%. As well, there are different formulations of HFCS with varying concentrations of fructose: beverages are 55% fructose ("HFCS-55"), for example, while baked goods are 42% ("HFCS-42").

While HFCS research is ongoing—and extremely high intakes of fructose can be problematic, though this is rare—for the average eater the bigger message is that sugar is sugar is sugar: there are 16 calories per teaspoon (4 g) and 48 per table-spoon, and overconsumption of *any* sugar can lead to deleterious cardiometabolic effects and weight gain. Whatever the name, whatever the source, most of us should cut way back. In fact, the World Health Organization (WHO) and the 2015–2020 Dietary Guidelines for Americans both recommend consuming no more than 10% of daily energy intake from sugar, adding that limiting it to 25 g daily (6 teaspoons) is even more beneficial.

What are the major fats and oils in our diet?

Fat is found in all cell membranes and plays a critical role in cell to cell communication throughout the body. It also cushions organs, provides insulation to maintain body temperature, and regulates genes involved in fat metabolism and inflammation. Fat also provides scrumptious flavors and textures to stimulate our palate, for better and for worse. Alongside carbohydrates, fat accounts for the largest percentage of calories in human diets. The proportion varies by personal preference and cultural norms: Mediterranean diets are high in fat, Japanese diets are low in fat, and typical American and British diets are in between. The majority of diets in the developing world are relatively low in fat and particularly high in carbohydrates, which are inexpensive, readily available, and less perishable.

Fat is the most energy-dense macronutrient, about 9 calories / g. Most of the fats in our diet are in the form of TGs, composed of glycerol and 3 fatty acids. TGs need to be digested into their in-dividual fatty acids ("free fatty acids") and glycerol in order to be absorbed. Fatty acids don't get as much attention as amino acids, but they will doubtless become better known to eaters like you in the coming decades given their diverse physiological effects. They have short, medium, long, or very long chains and may in-clude double bonds (unsaturated) or not (saturated); the bonds, in part, are what affects how they work in the body, that is, their bioactivity. Both short- and medium-chain fatty acids can cross the blood–brain barrier, just like glucose, and some medium-chain fatty acids play an important role in health by providing energy to colon cells. Long-chain and very long-chain fatty acids play critical roles throughout the body. Fat remains the victim of rampant misinformation, in part due to the 1980s low-fat-everything craze that deemed saturated fat and dietary cholesterol verboten. Cholesterol, for example, is a type of fat essential for many functions in the body, including synthesizing vitamin D and hormones. We make all the cholesterol we need and therefore do not need to consume it in our diet—though it's found in many animal foods like beef, dairy, and egg yolks. In the middle of the 20th century, cholesterol was thought to increase blood cholesterol, hence the risk of heart disease. But the science has evolved, and we now know there is little correlation between the cholesterol we get from diet and our blood cholesterol, much of which is under genetic control. Further, scientists now recognize that different fractions of cholesterol—like high-density lipoprotein ("good") cholesterol and low-density lipoprotein ("bad") cholesterol (HDL and LDL, respectively)—have different effects and are, in turn, responsive to various other foods and nutrients, like trans fat and refined carbohydrates. As a result, dietary cholesterol is no longer considered a risk factor for either high blood cholesterol or heart disease and is not part of the 2015–2020 Dietary Guidelines for Americans.

There are different kinds of fats, which have diverse physiological effects: all fat is not created equal. Thus, simply considering "total fat" is inadequate for today's informed eater seeking the healthiest choices. Saturated and unsaturated fats are the two main types, and unsaturated fats may be either monounsaturated (one double bond) or polyunsaturated (more than one double bond). Trans fat is a special type of unsaturated fat that acts like super-saturated fat in the body. Because polyunsaturated fats are often liquid at room temperature, they are often referred to as "oils."

How does saturated fat compare to unsaturated fat?

Saturated fatty acids (SFAs) have been a focal point of research for decades due to early studies suggesting that high intakes raised blood cholesterol, hence the risk of heart disease. As a result, eaters in the latter part of the 20th century cut their red meat consumption; increased chicken; and eschewed eggs, butter, and whole milk. Alas, the dietary recommendations encouraging decreasing sat fat as a way to reduce blood cholesterol and risk of heart disease were based on an incomplete understanding of the science, including the different components of blood cholesterol and the role of other fats. For example, we now know that total blood cholesterol is not as important in heart health as initially thought; it's the ratio of LDL and HDL that matters (and other properties of these lipoproteins that impact their role on atherogenesis and CVD). Genetics also impact cholesterol metabolism. While sat fat does lower LDL somewhat, it also decreases HDL—which means it doesn't have a particularly meaningful impact on the ratio.

Moreover, diet doesn't change in a vacuum, and if sat fat is being reduced, what is replacing it? Studies show clearly that swapping sat fat with quickly digested carbohydrates increases risk of heart disease by increasing LDL and blood triglycerides (TGs). Polyunsaturated fatty acids (PUFAs) are most protective, followed by monounsaturated fatty acids (MUFAs). A meta-analysis of 15 randomized controlled trials (RCTs), for instance, showed more than 25% reduced risk of cardiovascular events among those swapping SFAs for PUFAs.

Unsaturated fats can be recognized from their liquid state at room temperature, which is why they are sometimes called oils. They may have one double bond (MUFAs) or many (PUFAs). Oils are the major source of essential fatty acids in the diet and deliver vitamin E. Oils have the same calorie content as other fats—about 100–120 calories per tablespoon, depending on the type—but are heart-healthier due to their lack of saturation. Think, for example, about a solid fat like butter in comparison to a liquid fat like vegetable oil. The oil's fluidity contributes to its beneficial effect on the body, allowing cells to move with ease through our extensive network of bifurcated blood vessels and to communicate effectively with one another. Replacing digestible carbohydrates with unsaturated fats, particularly PUFAs, improves blood sugar control, insulin resistance, and insulin secretion, all of which protect against T2DM.

Is coconut oil a good choice? What about palm oil?

Coconut oil is a saturated vegetable oil, semisolid at room temperature. It is composed of 82% SFA, about half of which are medium-chain. Medium-chain fatty acids (specifically, lauric, myristic, and palmitic acids) have been shown to increase HDL in some animal experiments, and two small studies in 2003 found that providing overweight individuals with an oil made from 100% medium-chain fatty acids led to greater weight and fat loss (i.e., burned more fat) compared to those consuming oil made from 100% long-chain fatty acids. These studies led to headlines claiming coconut oil was a weight loss elixir, leading to a coconut craze despite its very high sat fat content—notwithstanding the fact that coconut oil, which is about 14% medium-chain fatty acids, is hardly the same as an oil made from 100% medium-chain fatty acids, which is what was tested. Since 2003, additional observational studies and RCTs in humans examined whether coconut oil led to favorable changes in weight and blood cholesterol but results were equivocal. Nevertheless, around 7 in 10 Americans thought coconut oil was nutritious when surveyed in 2017.

There is considerable evidence that coconut oil does in fact lead to increases in HDL, as do most fats. But it also increases LDL, thus having a negligible effect on the ratio, like other saturated fats. Moreover, some RCTs showed that coconut oil raised LDL compared to both PUFA-rich safflower oil and MUFA-rich olive oil.

In aggregate, the relationship between coconut oil and weight loss requires more research studies in humans, while its effects on LDL are well appreciated. Therefore, WHO and the current Dietary Guidelines for Americans still recommend limiting saturated fat (which includes coconut oil) to no more than 10% of daily calories. Although no RCTs have specifically examined how coconut oil compares to PUFA- and MUFA-rich vegetable oils on CVD directly, like having a heart attack, the American Heart Association 2017 guidelines specifically advised against consuming coconut oil due to its role in raising LDL and instead continued recommending swapping SFAs for PUFAs and MUFAs. Thus, while coconut fruit and its oil may play an innocuous role when consumed in moderation as part of an energy-balanced diet—just like butter and cheese and other foods high in sat fat—choosing unsaturated fats as your go-to oils is far more likely to promote healthy cholesterol levels that keep your heart happy.

Palm oil has a similar chemistry to coconut oil: its major fatty acid is palmitic acid,[1] which is medium-chain. It is more shelf-stable than unsaturated vegetable oils and is used in about half of consumer products worldwide, according to the World Wildlife Fund (WWF); it is ubiquitous in processed foods like cookies, snacks, and crackers. Like coconut oil, palm oil is not the best choice for heart health as it doesn't provide the same beneficial effects on blood cholesterol or TGs as unsaturated fats like soybean and canola oils.

There are also grave social and environmental concerns with palm oil production, including monoculture and deforestation that threatens several endangered species (e.g., orangutans) and child and forced labor. The industry is also renowned for utilizing banned pesticides and exploiting farmworkers. Many of these offenses were cited in a 2016 Amnesty International report titled "The Great Palm Oil Scandal: Labour Abuse Behind Big Brand Names." Yet consumer awareness is often shrouded by vague ingredient labels: "vegetable oil" or "palmityl alcohol" may be used rather than "palm oil," for instance.[2] Conscious eaters can avoid foods made with palm oil by looking to the WWF, which lists products made from palm oil on its website. The Roundtable on Sustainable Palm Oil (RSPO) label and "Green Palm Sustainability" are also helpful, though they haven't always reflected sound practices that protect both planet and people.

What are omega-3 and omega-6 fatty acids?

There are two classes of essential fatty acids (EFAs): omega-3 (aka, n-3) and omega-6 (aka, n-6). They cannot be synthesized by the diet and must be consumed in the diet. Both are incorporated into cell membranes throughout the body. EFAs are also precursors to eicosanoids, compounds that play critical functions such as controlling inflammation. Inflammation wreaks havoc throughout the body and has been associated with a higher risk of heart disease, obesity, arthritis, dementia, renal disease, and acute pancreatitis.

Three major n-3s are eicosapentaenoic acid (EPA), docosahexaenoic acid (DHA), and alpha-linolenic acid (ALA). ALA is found in vegetable oils, walnuts, and flax seeds, as well as some leafy greens and grass-fed animals. EPA and DHA are very long-chain because of their many carbon molecules, which lead to special actions in the body; they are often called "marine fatty acids" as they are only found in fish, algae, and, to a smaller degree, sea vegetables. Marine fatty acids are particularly beneficial for eye, brain, and heart health. DHA is so vital to vision and cognition, including in utero, that pregnant women are encouraged to consume seafood (Chapter 13). And DHA, which occurs naturally in breast milk, has been added to infant formula for the past several decades in the US and other countries because of its critical role in infancy. ALA has many fewer carbon molecules and, while still beneficial, doesn't play the same role as DHA and EPA. Although it can be lengthened in the body, the process is inefficient: only about 10% of ALA is converted to EPA or DHA, on average.

EPA and DHA (and their major sources, seafood, Chapter 13) have been related to lower blood pressure and heart rate, lower TGs, less atherosclerosis, and improved insulin resistance. For these reasons, the American Heart Association recommends eating 2 servings of seafood per week to obtain sufficient EPA and DHA and 1 serving daily for those with heart disease. The role of fish oil supplements in the prevention of cardiometabolic events has thus been a major topic of investigation for the past several decades. Though many observational studies show favorable effects, evidence from RCTs is less consistent.

Omega-3s from both diet and supplements have also been examined in conditions ranging from dementia to depression, Crohn's to colitis, T2DM to cancer. Results remain intriguing but inconclusive in most of these diseases. Normal aging reduces DHA in brain tissue, and individuals suffering from Alzheimer's disease have particularly low DHA, for example. Some animal and observational studies of cognitive decline, dementias, and Alzheimer's suggest a protective effect, especially in those with early Alzheimer's. In major depressive disorder, a recent meta-analysis of 20 RCTs found that n-3s had only small to modest benefits for depressive symptoms.

The second class of EFA is omega-6 (n-6), primarily consumed in the diet as alpha-linoleic acid, which is then converted into arachidonic acid (ARA). Like EPA and DHA, ARA is also found in cell membranes and has eicosanoid action relevant for moderating inflammation and immune responses. ARA plays a critical role in infant development and is thus also added to baby formula alongside

DHA. Many Western diets are very high in linoleic acid, hence ARA, mainly because it's found in the vegetable oils used in so many processed foods. At the same time, diets are often quite low in EPA and DHA. Those with diets low in n-3 have more n-6 in their cell membranes. This has been hypothesized to cause more inflammation, suggesting that the n-3/n-6 ratio is important for health. The science is not conclusive, but what is known for certain is that both classes are essential.

What is trans fat?

Trans fats occur naturally in ruminant animals like cows and sheep, so people who consume those foods will always get a small bit in their diets. Yet the vast majority of trans fats are industrially produced, in which they are chemically altered through the addition of hydrogen—"partially hydrogenated"—to be solid and more shelf-stable. This is how unsaturated fats like canola oil are converted into "partially hydrogenated" fats like margarine.

Procter & Gamble was the first to use trans fat in a food product. Launched in 1911, Crisco is a shelf-stable and less expensive alternative to animal fats like butter and lard. It grew in popularity due to its performance in home baking and frying. Margarine sales soared in the 1940s because butter was rationed during World War II. As the 20th century progressed, studies began showing an association between fat and heart disease, leading the American Heart Association to launch in 1957 its first campaign directed toward decreasing fat consumption. In part due to consumer demands in the 1980s, fast food restaurants began using partially hydrogenated oils, particularly in frying. Scientists began examining trans fat and reached a scientific consensus at the end of the 20th century that they were a major contributor to atherogenesis and heart disease. A movement emerged to remove trans fats from the food industry, beginning with Denmark in 2004 and continuing in many countries thereafter as recommended by WHO. Trans fat was added to food labels in the US in 2006, and in 2007 New York became the first state to ban its use in restaurants. The food industry later began voluntarily removing trans fat from foods across the board. Most trans fat has been removed from the food supply in the US and many other high-income countries, although policies and practices are still catching up in the developing world. In 2018, WHO urged all nations to ban trans fats, which are thought to kill 500 000 people annually.

Is fat "fattening"? Are low-fat foods healthy?

Fat has been in the spotlight for decades, with thousands of studies examining its role in weight due to its high calorie content and palatability: it's delicious, which can stimulate overconsumption. Moreover, fat is more likely to be stored in adipose (fat) tissue compared to protein and carbohydrate. A 2010 comprehensive literature review found that whether dietary fat is truly "fattening," however, depends on different factors. In energy-deficit conditions, like a low-calorie weight loss diet, RCTs have found that high-fat diets led to *greater* weight loss than low-fat diets. This is due to ketosis, in which the body "burns" fat for energy when inadequate carbs are consumed, thus promoting fat oxidation and weight loss. In other words, when we eat carbs, the body will use those first to fuel our everyday metabolism and activities; it's only when carbs are restricted that the body will use fat instead, including that eaten and, if needed, stored. This is what leads to fat loss in, say, the Atkins (low-carb, high-fat) diet. Conversely, low-fat diets have also been shown to promote weight loss in studies where people follow their own diet plan, assuming a negative calorie balance (i.e., calories in are less than calories out).

Still, excess calories from any source will lead to weight gain if they exceed energy expenditure—and any diet can facilitate weight loss as long as calories are cut. One size doesn't fit all, and creating a health-giving diet for life is the key, whether it's high-fat or low-fat (Chapter 17). And remembering that some fats—and some carbs—are more healthful than others when it comes to chronic disease prevention is paramount. There are bounteous low- and nonfat options on supermarket shelves, for example, including cookies, chips, cheese, ice cream, deli meats, and beyond—not to mention the still-popular frozen yogurt. These foods often provide fewer calories, but fats are often replaced with quickly digested carbs that spike blood sugar. And low- and nonfat salad dressings are often less nutritious than their full-fat cousins that include healthful

PUFAs and MUFAs, albeit lower in calories. Plus, there are plenty of situations where low- and nonfat alternatives help reduce saturated fat intakes (like reduced fat and skim milk) and control calories. Reading the nutrition facts panel and ingredient lists will facilitate an informed choice.

Why are protein and amino acids important?

Animal foods come to mind when people think of protein, whether pork or beef, chicken or goat, seafood or insects, eggs or dairy. Yet protein is found in both animal and plant foods and, like carbohydrates and fats, includes carbon, hydrogen, and oxygen. Protein is the only macronutrient that includes nitrogen, however; and its unique side chains and chemistry define its function (much like the individual fatty acids that make up a triglyceride). There are some 25 000 proteins encoded in the human genome, which create a "dynamic system of structural and functional elements that exchange nitrogen with the environment."

Proteins provide about 4 calories/g, like carbohydrates, and are composed of varying amounts of amino acids (remember that grade-school biology mantra "amino acids are the building blocks of protein"?), usually around 20. Proteins are in a constant cycle of breakdown and synthesis in the body, creating a pool of amino acids able to meet the body's specific physiological needs. When we eat protein, it is digested into its amino acids and component tripeptides and dipeptides (smaller protein byproducts). Amino acids are further broken down in the liver into alpha-keto acids, which can be drawn upon for energy or resynthesized into other amino acids to suit the body's needs. Nitrogen-containing urea, the major byproduct of protein metabolism, travels through the blood from the liver to the kidney, where it is filtered and excreted through urine or reabsorbed if needed. The filtration rate increases in relation to protein intake and can strain poorly functioning kidneys (like those with renal disease), though healthy kidneys generally adjust to a range of protein intakes.

More than a century of research has led to a rich body of knowledge regarding protein and amino acid biochemistry, including digestibility, bioavailability, and utilization. Many different techniques have been created to measure protein quality as a result; animal products usually come out on top, although soy ranks as high as beef with one method. Nonetheless, a 2007 WHO report concluded that differences in protein quality are small and may be far less meaningful to health than originally reported from early studies: humans are adaptive in utilizing protein, regardless of source. Excessive protein intake can negatively impact liver and bone health as well as those with kidney disease, though the evidence is still evolving as to the long-term effect in healthy adults. A larger problem is obesity: excess protein, like other macronutrients, will be stored as fat in adipose tissue.

Amino acids include sulfur as well as nitrogen, essential for multifarious functions throughout the body, including creating enzymes to catalyze chemical reactions; providing strength and structure to muscles, skin, and hair; transporting oxygen to all cells and organs; and building a healthy immune system. Inadequate dietary protein severely compromises growth and development, decreases ability to fight infection and disease, and is ultimately fatal. The human body can synthesize many of the amino acids it needs for critical body functions by recycling unused proteins. These amino acids—alanine, arginine, asparagine, aspartic acid, cysteine, glutamic acid, glutamine, glycine, proline, selenocysteine, serine, and tyrosine—are thus considered nonessential. (Arginine, cysteine, glutamine, proline, selenocysteine, serine, and tyrosine may become essential if sufficient precursors aren't available to enable synthesis.) Additional amino acids can only be obtained through the diet and are considered essential—histidine, isoleucine, leucine, lysine, methionine, phenylalanine, threonine, tryptophan, and valine—just like some fatty acids.

Some amino acids are recognizable to eaters. Tryptophan gets attention each Thanksgiving to explain turkey's soporific effects—although it's an urban myth as sleepiness is most likely due to eating mounds of food, not tryptophan per se. Phenylketonuria (i.e., PKU) is a rare genetic disease that causes phenylalanine to build up in the body, and newborns in many countries are tested at birth to successfully manage the disease. Glutamic acid is one of the most abundant amino acids, and its salt, glutamate, is responsible for the umami taste found in foods like cheese, seaweed, fermented foods (e.g., soy sauce), yeast, and tomatoes. Monosodium glutamate (MSG) is the salt of glutamic acid, synthesized in 1908 by Japanese biochemist

Kikunae Ikeda to duplicate the savory goodness of kombu, a type of seaweed. It has been used as a flavor enhancer, particularly in Asian cuisine, and has been approved for use in the EU, US, and many other countries since the mid-20th century. MSG remains associated with "Chinese restaurant syndrome," but reviews of well-designed studies with adequate controls have concluded that no true association between MSG and headaches exists. (A similar conclusion was reached regarding associations with asthma, although data are limited.) While specific amino acids receive more research (and media) attention than others, remembering each one isn't something most eaters need to consider: consuming a varied diet will ensure adequate intake, and significant changes in scientific understanding relevant for disease prevention will lead to public health action when necessary.

Protein-containing foods are sometimes classified as either "complete" (containing all of the essential amino acids) or "incomplete" (lacking one or more essential amino acids), though the concept is outdated. Animal foods contain "complete" proteins, while most plant foods do not, with a few exceptions (e.g., quinoa, buckwheat, soy, hemp, chia, potato). Legumes are low in cysteine, tryptophan, and methionine, for example, while grains lack lysine. A rice and bean bowl thus contains "complementary proteins," a classic example of "protein combining" designed to create a complete protein. Newer science indicates there is no need for vegetarians to create a complete protein at every meal from sundry plant foods (happily), as long as all essential amino acids are obtained throughout the day. Furthermore, the body is able to "complete" proteins on its own in many cases through its pool of amino acids. Consuming a varied diet with adequate calories often ensures that needs are met—without memorizing lists of essential amino acids, remembering which foods contain what, or creating "complete" proteins at each meal.

Like other macronutrient studies, much protein research today is focused on chronic disease prevention. Such studies are arguably more difficult to conduct given that humans are generally adept at managing protein needs; and protein consumption is, on average, less variable than fat and carbohydrate intake. There is some evidence that plant proteins are associated with lower LDL and a decreased risk of CVD, though such studies are often confounded by other aspects of the diet, like intakes of other protective nutrients and foods that occur alongside higher plant protein intakes. A bigger issue is the general overconsumption of protein, on average about 100 g daily for American adults, most of which comes from animal foods. Protein-rich animal foods are often bundled with saturated fat and, in the case of red and processed meat, a host of elements that increase the risk of cancer (Chapter 4). Food production of such protein sources also strains environmental resources and compromises sustainability (Chapter 12).

How much protein do we require, and do some people need more than others?

We need protein daily as we lose nitrogen through sweat, urine, and feces as well as skin cells, hair, and nails. Heightened periods of growth and development raise protein needs, such as pregnancy, infancy, lactation, and early childhood, as do sickness and infection, which increase immune responses and tissue recovery (like a burn requiring collagen for rebuilding skin).

More than a century of nitrogen balance studies have been performed to determine human protein and amino acid needs, which are periodically reviewed and updated. The most recent WHO report (2007) concluded that 0.83 g/kg of body weight per day (133 mg nitrogen daily) safely met the requirements of most adults. Accordingly, European and American guidelines both recommend 0.8 g/kg of body weight, about 8 g for every 20 pounds (or, multiply your weight in pounds by 0.36); the UK recommendation is similar (0.75 g/kg). This equates to about 56 g daily for adult men and 46 for women (71 if pregnant or breastfeeding). Like carbohydrate and fat, dietary guidelines provide a range of acceptable intakes consistent with good health. The Institute of Medicine, for example, recommends that daily protein as a percentage of energy should range between 10% and 35%, leaving room for individuals to create a diet that suits different food preferences and lifestyles.

Protein has come into the dietary spotlight, perhaps due to the still-present fear of fat and confusion about whether carbohydrates like grains are nutritious (Chapter 10). Many people are piling on the protein, whether in fortified snacks or as part of a meat-centric Paleo diet (Chapter 3). Protein is powerful: it's necessary for life, like fat and carbohydrate. It also provides the greatest satiety due to its role in helping release chemicals from the small intestine that help us feel full. That same feeling tends to last longer than a carbohydrate-rich meal, prolonging our satiation (continuing to feel satisfied after we stop eating). These properties are indeed important and have boosted protein's presence on our plates as a weight management strategy.

That said, the notion of "needing more protein" is misplaced, at best. Americans and Europeans generally consume far more protein than needed, infants to elderly, particularly American men. A closer look at the sources of protein in the diet is also informative. The majority of Americans consume more meat, poultry, and eggs and less seafood than recommended for preventing chronic diseases. Many also do not turn to plant-based proteins like beans, nuts, and seeds. Further, many protein-rich snacks packed into purses are loaded in sugar and sodium and, in some cases, refined grains, making them less than optimal for health—especially given our dismal intake of vegetables and fruit. And Americans aren't the only ones consuming more protein than they need, either. The World Resources Institute shows that people across the world, on every continent, consume more protein than required—and plant protein intakes almost always fall short in places with higher incomes.

There are, however, some who do have higher protein needs than others. Some elite athletes are actively involved in building and breaking down muscle, and bodybuilders in particular benefit from extra protein to develop muscle mass and strength. Protein is also important for optimal muscle recovery following prolonged exercise. The specific amounts needed vary by sport, age, weight, sex, and exercise intensity. These recommendations do not pertain to kids on a soccer field, high school athletes, or even extremely active adults, whose activity level does not rival those of professional athletes and, hence, do not have higher protein needs than their peers. The human body is an amazing machine that adapts to a wide array of metabolic conditions to ensure a healthy nitrogen balance.

Nonetheless, newer evidence is emerging to suggest that adults involved in regular weight training may benefit from higher protein intake. A 2017 meta-analysis and systematic review of 49 RCTs found that those supplementing their diet with additional protein

from any source (liquid or solid, vegan or animal)—total
1.6 g/kg—showed about 10% greater strength and m
Effects increased with training experience but decrease
These results are intriguing but do not pertain to the majority oι
(sedentary) adults.

Whether current protein recommendations are adequate to meet
the needs of older adults is an active area of investigation, as rates
of synthesis are lower in this age group and other biological and
lifestyle changes with aging lead to a loss of lean mass. A growing
body of research is showing that higher protein intake is needed
to retain muscle and bone mass, which helps maintain mobility
and reduce frailty, falls, and mortality. Evenly distributed protein
across meals and throughout the day may also be beneficial, particularly when accompanied by resistance training. A small meta-
analysis of 7 prospective observational studies also indicated that
increasing protein intake may protect against stroke. Due to these
and other studies, one international study group recently suggested
that adults aged 65 and older should consume 1.0–1.3 g/kg of body
weight daily and that those with chronic diseases (except kidney
disease, which requires limiting protein intake) may need as much
as 1.5 g/kg daily.

Some national guidelines do advise higher protein intakes for
older adults, including the Ministry of Health for Australia and
New Zealand, which recommends 1.07 g/kg for men and 0.94 g/
kg for women older than 70 years. Yet protein recommendations
do not differ by age in the US, EU, and Canada. The fact remains,
however, that while guidelines are important, they do not reflect
intake: the majority of people already consume a great deal more
protein than recommended, and it's coming from the wrong places
(i.e., it is too reliant on meat and processed meat). And there are
few studies looking at long-term risks of excess protein intake. High
intake is particularly problematic for those with impaired kidney
function, as noted—and the National Kidney Foundation warns that
1 in 3 Americans are at risk for kidney impairment because of high
blood pressure or diabetes. There are also a few studies that suggest
that high protein intake later in life, particularly animal protein, can
lead to cancer, a result of its effects on increasing cell multiplication,
though more research is needed.

Do high-protein diets lead to greater weight loss and improved cardiovascular health?

Though the putative role of high-protein diets in health and weight had been around for decades, the close of the 20th century saw renewed interest in "Atkins"-style diets, leading to the high-protein/low-carb backlash of the aughts. As mentioned, protein is the most satiating nutrient, which is why protein-rich foods are helpful in managing appetite and controlling calories. A number of RCTs initially showed a greater amount of weight loss among those consuming high-protein diets compared to low-fat/high-carb diets. High-protein diets do indeed lead to faster initial weight loss, in part because water is necessary to metabolize protein. Therefore, much of the initial loss is water weight, not body fat. Additional studies following people for longer time periods showed that those on high-protein diets experienced similar weight loss over time. Since then, numerous systematic reviews and meta-analyses have compared various isoenergetic diets (i.e., equal calories) on weight loss and cardiovascular health and have found little difference in weight loss, blood pressure, LDL, HDL total cholesterol, triglycerides, and fasting blood glucose after one or two years of follow-up. Thus, the state of the science is that *any* diet can lead to weight loss and improved cardiovascular outcomes, as long as calories are in a negative balance. A key is finding a weight loss diet that works where adherence can be sustained and weight loss can be maintained. (See also Chapter 17.)

Part IV

FOOD, GLORIOUS FOOD

Everything we eat is based on food of some kind, vegetable or animal, which in turn includes a wide array of nutritious elements—and other things, too—that impact our health and longevity. How food is produced also has implications for farmworkers, the environment, and society as a whole: it's not just about you.

9

CREATING A COLORFUL PLATE

VEGETABLES AND FRUITS

How do vegetables differ nutritionally?

Botanically, vegetables are the edible parts of plants and, thus, technically include fruits (the seed-containing, mature ovary). Vegetables are mainly carbohydrates, including starch, nonstarch polysaccharides, and fibers with varying levels of vitamins C, K, E, B_6, thiamin, niacin, and folate and minerals potassium, copper, magnesium, iron, manganese, and choline. There are many different ways to categorize vegetables, including color, an indicator of phytochemical content (Chapter 7), nutrient composition, and culinary use, which is why some botanical fruits are considered vegetables, like tomatoes. Leaves and roots of the same plant species differ in nutrient content, which isn't surprising given their biological functions: roots provide energy for growth and are high in carbohydrates while leaves offer plentiful vitamins and minerals due to their active role in photosynthesis and other metabolic processes.

Common vegetable groups and the examples below begin with the US Department of Agriculture (USDA) scheme and break out additional categories based on current nutrition research; sea vegetables are singled out because of their prominence in Asian diets (Chapter 17) and increasing popularity in the West.

- **Dark green:** Spinach, grape leaves, kale, greens (beet/collard/turnip), and broccoli; rich in vitamin K, lutein, and water; many are sources of calcium.

- **Red and orange:** Winter squash, sweet potato, carrot, tomato, and bell peppers; rich in carotenoids.

- **Cruciferous:** Cabbage, cauliflower, broccoli, Brussels sprouts, radish, turnip, bok choy, kale, greens, kohlrabi, rutabaga, horseradish, wasabi, and arugula; rich in glucosinolates.

- **Starchy:** Potato, corn, plantain, water chestnut, jicama, and green peas; higher in calories, digestible carbohydrate, and potassium compared to other vegetables, though each has unique benefits (e.g., corn provides resistant starch and ranks higher than any other vegetable on total antioxidant content).

- **Allium:** Onion, leek, garlic, shallot, chive, and scallion; rich in organo-sulfur compounds and quercetin, a flavonoid antioxidant.

- **Other:** Avocado, olive, mushroom, okra, beet, cucumber, cactus, summer squash, eggplant, string and long beans, celery, and bamboo shoots have varied nutrient compositions unique from other groups; iceberg lettuce, celery, and cucumber are mainly water with few notable nutrients; avocado is rich in monounsaturated fat; eggplant is high in fiber and has a unique purple phytochemical named nasunin.

- **Sea vegetables (aka, seaweed):** Three major varieties include green algae (~7000 species, e.g., sea lettuce, sea grapes), brown algae (~4000 species; e.g., kombu/kelp, wakame, hijiki), and red algae (~2000 species; e.g., nori, agar-agar, and dulse); iodine powerhouses that also include vitamin C, manganese, vitamin B_2, vitamin A, copper, calcium, potassium, fiber, omega-3 docasahexaenoic acid (DHA), and iron; unique polysaccharides contain sulfur (called fucoidans); rich in antioxidant polyphenols (e.g., carotenoids and flavonoids).

- **Herbs and spices:** Include miniscule quantities of a range of phytochemicals (e.g., flavonoids, phenols, alkaloids, and tannins), vitamins, and minerals.

Some vegetable (and fruit) skins are thin (e.g., carrot, radish, summer squash, cucumber), others are more fibrous (e.g., eggplant, potato), and several have tough outer rinds that are virtually indigestible (winter squash, pumpkin). Yet the skins of many not only are edible but provide nutrients, texture, and flavor to food while reducing food waste and saving food dollars. A few examples include carrots, cucumbers, all potatoes, eggplant, and delicata squash. While pesticide residue can remain on vegetable skins, a hearty scrub will remove most, and there is no evidence to show that residues confer a health risk; the benefits of consuming the whole plant likely outweigh any potential adverse effect. Likewise, there is no need to follow "raw food" fads (Chapter 4): the best thing you can do is eat *more*, however prepared. (Except deep-fried, which should be enjoyed only in moderation, alas—as you already knew).

What's special about herbs and spices?

Herbs and spices play a distinctive role in both culinary traditions and herbal medicine. Herbs are generally considered the leaves from aromatic plants grown in temperate regions and can be enjoyed fresh or dried. Spices come from the roots, seeds, bark, berries, or flower buds of tropical plants and are most frequently consumed dried, though some are also eaten fresh (e.g., ginger, turmeric). Herbs and spices have no calories and are generally used in small amounts to give foods flavor, aroma, and color.

While the health benefits of herbs and spices have been appreciated for millennia, they have only recently garnered scientific attention. Individual studies and a handful of randomized controlled trials (RCTs) have shown that herbs and spices have a range of biological activities related to the development of cancer (turmeric, saffron, mustard, bay leaf, garlic, ginger, turmeric, and mustard seeds) and cardiovascular disease (CVD) (cinnamon, ginger, garlic, turmeric, red pepper, and fenugreek), among other health conditions. (A free herbs and spices fact sheet is available at pknewby.com.) Intriguingly, a dietary database of 3100 foods found that traditional herbal medicines had the highest antioxidant content, and spices and herbs were second.

A number of studies show enhanced effects when herbs and spices are consumed together (e.g., a supplement including both curcuminoids found in turmeric and piperine found in black pepper). Studies of traditional herbal medicines individually and in combination also show promising results. Two retrospective studies in Taiwan found that patients with type 2 diabetes mellitus (T2DM) who used Chinese herbal medicine in addition to conventional medical treatment had improved survival from hypertension and stroke compared to those who didn't, for instance.

Current evidence is inadequate to support dietary guidelines for specific herbs and spices, though today's "natural" food stores are replete with concoctions touting too-good-to-be-true effects (usually). Buyer beware: the supplement industry is fraught with weak regulations and numerous incidents of mislabeling and adulteration, rendering many products not only useless but, in rare cases, dangerous. But there's no reason not to spice up your life: these little plants boost nutrition and add lively flavor to your diet. And, in the future, scientific research may support the age-old wisdom espousing the disease-preventing, health-promoting effects of herbs and spices—and modern pharmaceuticals will follow suit by including them in tomorrow's medicines.

What are the various kinds of fruit?

The bright colors and intoxicating aromas of fruit have long attracted those in the animal kingdom, including, eventually, human primates. This symbiotic relationship nourishes consumers and sustains the plant species by disseminating the seeds. At the same time, these same hues and fragrances act as deterrents to pests and predators, protection that enables successful reproduction and self-preservation.

Fruits are generally rich in carbohydrates, including fiber; vitamins C, A, and K; water; minerals potassium and magnesium; and an array of phytochemicals that vary by species. The seeds of many fruits can be toxic due to their cyanogenic glycosides—think cyanide—though loads would need to be consumed to deliver ill effects. Vitamin C acts as a powerful antioxidant throughout the body, as do many other phytochemicals. Fruit is higher in simple sugars like glucose, sucrose, and fructose than most other food groups; some also contain sorbitol, a sugar alcohol. However, most have a low glycemic index (i.e., impact on blood sugar) because of the other nutrients they contain, like fiber, water, and minerals. Common fruit groups follow.

- **Citrus:** Orange, grapefruit, lemon, lime, tangerine, and clementine are rich in vitamin C and fiber; red and pink grapefruit have the antioxidant lycopene but also furanocoumarins, phytochemicals that interact dangerously with more than 40 drugs.

- **Berries:** Blueberry, blackberry, strawberry, cranberry, and grapes are rich in vitamin C, manganese, and copper and are among the top sources of antioxidant and anti-inflammatory phytochemicals in the diet, particularly anthocyanins. Strawberries provide flavonoids and phenolic acids, while blueberries and grapes provide vitamin K.

- **Melons:** Watermelon, honeydew, cantaloupe, musk, and other varieties are especially high in water. Orange melons have a more diverse array of nutrients than many other fruits, including provitamin A carotenoids as well as potassium, copper, magnesium, folate, and several B vitamins; watermelon provides lycopene as well as citrulline, an amino acid.

- **Cored fruits:** Apple and pear are rich in anthocyanins and total dietary fiber, particularly pectin, a soluble fiber facilitating satiety.

- **Stone fruits:** Peach, plum, nectarine, apricot, and cherry are powerhouses of vitamin C, carotenoids, fiber, and potassium; apricots lead the pack.

- **Tropical fruits:** Banana, pomegranate, mango, guava, kiwi (Chinese gooseberry), pineapple, papaya, fig, lychee, date, jackfruit, breadfruit, and coconut are diverse in nutrients. Bananas boast potassium; kiwi provides vitamins C and A and copper; and coconut provides vitamin C, iron, and magnesium as well as saturated and monounsaturated fatty acids (and about 350 calories for one-quarter of a fresh, medium drupe).

The sugar content of fruit varies; thus, some have a greater impact on blood sugar than others, like any other sweet food. Dried fruit is nutrient-rich but quite energy-dense and particularly high in sugar since the water has been removed. One cup of dried apricots has about 310 calories compared to about 80 in a cup of fresh, for instance. Fruit juice is the opposite: it's all liquid, a quickly consumed sugar and calorie boost that often lacks the fiber content of fresh, canned, frozen, or dried fruit. For example, pomegranate seeds (arils) provide 70 calories in one-half cup (87 g); there are around 130 calories per cup when ground into juice, and the fiber is often removed. (See Chapter 16 for juicing.) The American Diabetes Association reminds that diabetics (both type 1 and type 2) can still enjoy fruit, especially whole fruit, assuming it's part of a diet that closely monitors blood sugar.

When it comes to disease prevention, are some vegetables and fruits better than others?

Today, each fruit and vegetable (group) has its own rich literature—pear to persimmon, squash to sweet potato—critically important in advancing knowledge about how specific plants contribute to health. Many fruits and veggies have come in and out of fashion; some are touted as the "superfood" of the day. (Kale, anyone?) A detailed discussion of each is far beyond the space of this book, though a few examples are described below.

The vibrant colors of **berries** reflect rich phytochemical content that, together with their vitamins and minerals, contribute to anti-inflammatory effects. Berries also contain mighty antioxidants, among the highest concentration across fruit groups. Pomegranates, blueberries, raspberries, and strawberries have been shown to reduce arthritis pain and inflammation in some studies. And a 2018 review of RCTs found promising evidence that both blueberries and cranberries helped those with T2DM maintain healthy blood sugar levels. Jewel-colored cranberries have shown cardioprotective benefits as well as "anticancer, antimutagenic, antimicrobial, anti-inflammatory, and anti-neurodegenerative properties." Cranberries have been most studied in relation to urinary tract infections (UTIs). While many experiments show beneficial effects, particularly in laboratory and in vitro models at high doses, a recent review of 24 studies concluded that cranberries (whole berries, juice, etc.) did not significantly reduce UTI symptoms. This could be because the dose of the bioactive components in cranberries was insufficient or there really is no effect. While UTI research will continue, there is no downside to eating cranberries, one of many healthful berries.

Often overlooked, everyday **apples** have much to offer nutrition-ally—and are easier on the wallet than many other fruits. Laboratory studies indicate that apples' myriad phytochemicals may play a role in the reduced risk of several cancers, CVD, and asthma and might also have beneficial effects on cognitive decline and normal aging (including Alzheimer's), diabetes, weight management, and bone and gastrointestinal health. Among other mechanisms, apples' polyphenols reach the large intestine relatively intact, where they favorably impact gut bacteria (Chapter 4). Research also shows that those consuming apples have higher-quality diets and are less likely to become overweight.[1]

Crucifers are unique due to their high concentrations of glucosinolates, which are metabolized into isothiocyanates, sulfur-containing compounds that have antioxidant and anti-inflammatory activity and are involved in modulating "detox" enzymes that elim-inate carcinogens from the body. Many epidemiologic studies have shown that cruciferous veggies may protect against cancers of the colon, lung, prostate, breast, bladder, and kidney. A meta-analysis and systematic review of 33 studies observed a 16% lower odds of colon cancer among cruciferous vegetable consumers. Broccoli was particularly effective at reducing the risk of colorectal neoplasms, by 20%. Importantly, these studies have also revealed important gene–diet interactions, which will be helpful in personalizing nutrition recommendations in future years.

On the other hand, some vegetables get a bad rap, like **white potatoes**. While this a staple of many traditional diets and provide vitamins, minerals, fiber, and phytochemicals, potatoes are also quite starchy and have a high glycemic index (GI, Chapter 8), a risk factor for T2DM. Observational studies show equivocal associations between potatoes (baked, mashed, boiled, fried, etc.) and health outcomes ranging from T2DM to obesity, though no RCTs have been performed. A systematic review of 13 studies found consistent relationships only between French fries and obesity or T2DM, al-though only when more than 2–3 servings per week were consumed. Findings may be attributable not to the fries per se but to their cal-orie content (alongside their delectable dipping sauces), as well as how they contribute to the overall dietary pattern. Importantly, the GI of a potato depends on how it's cooked and served: potatoes can be part of a healthy diet in moderation but contain more calories and fewer phytochemicals than many other vegetables. Relying on potatoes as your main vegetable, especially French fries, is not the optimal recipe for health—which you probably already knew.

Sea vegetables (aka, seaweed or algae) also deserve a shout out. They've played a role in Asian diets (notably, in Japan, China, and Korea) for more than 10 000 years and were also a part of traditional diets in northern coastal regions of places like Norway, Ireland, Wales, and Nova Scotia. Seaweed contains a wide collection of nutrients and phytonutrients found in ocean environments that can't be found anywhere else. They are low in calories and high in fiber, and their unique polysaccharides containing sulfur ("sulfated polysaccharides") have shown antioxidant, antiviral, and anticoagulant properties. They also demonstrate anticancer activity in laboratory and human studies. Sea vegetables play a major role in the diets of Okinawans, one of the world's longest-lived populations (Chapter 17). And algae can play an important function in vegetarian diets that lack seafood, boosting essential omega-3 fatty acid DHA intake, critical for health and development (Chapter 8).

How much vegetables and fruit are we eating, and why should we consume more, of all kinds?

USDA first called out vegetables and fruit in 1916 and began emphasizing specific types as early as 1930. The Dietary Guidelines for Americans, issued every 5 years since 1980, has been emphasizing, "Choose a diet with plenty of vegetables and fruit" since 1990. Today, the 2015–2020 guidelines state, "Healthy eating patterns include a variety of vegetables and fruit." Thus, despite the oft-heard claim that "nutritionists are always changing their minds," many fundamental messages have been around for more than a century. While science continues to uncover ever more reasons to eat your fruits and vegetables from potent phytochemicals to diet–gene interactions, research showing the profound impact of produce on health is not new—and neither is dietary advice encouraging consumption.

Yet, only 10% of Americans meet daily recommendations for vegetables and 15% for fruit (1–3½ cups and 1–2½ cups, respectively, depending on age and sex). Moreover, *Homo sapiens* are creatures of habit, relying mainly on carrots and tomatoes, apples and oranges, rather than choosing a colorful array of plants offering richly varied nutritional benefits (and flavors!). White potatoes are most common, comprising 25% of total vegetable consumption among Americans on average and 28–35% among children 2–18 years old. Intakes of dark green, red and orange, and cruciferous veggies are particularly low, while vegetables like iceberg lettuce and cucumbers dominate the "other" group.

Nutrition scientists around the world agree that the insufficient quantity and limited variety of vegetables and fruits consumed are contributors to diet-related chronic diseases, and greater health benefits are often observed at levels beyond the ubiquitous "5 a day" message in the US. There is little, if any, downside to consuming copious vegetables and fruits for health protection, especially when they supplant energy-dense foods high in sugar, refined carbohydrates, and calories. Many studies show a somewhat more protective effect of vegetables in certain diseases (e.g., liver disease, some cancers), likely due in part to the much larger variety of phytochemicals among veggies alongside the lower calorie and sugar content. It's for this reason that many scientists today emphasize "vegetables and fruit" rather than "fruit and vegetables."

Indeed, there are thousands of studies in vitro and in vivo alongside observational studies, animal studies, meta-analyses, and systematic reviews showing the health-protective, disease-preventive effects of consuming produce. A 2017 analysis of 95 prospective cohort studies, for instance, found that for each 200-g intake of vegetables and fruits consumed daily there is an 8% risk reduction in coronary heart disease (CHD) and CVD, a 16% risk reduction in stroke, and a 3% risk reduction in any cancer. Death from any cause was 10% lower for each 200 g consumed. Higher intakes compared with lower intakes (<40 g daily) showed greater risk reduction: those consuming 800 g daily (around 10 servings) had 24%, 33%, 28%, and 31% reductions in CHD, stroke, CVD, and all-cause mortality, respectively, compared to those consuming 500 g daily (around 6 servings) at 16%, 28%, 22%, and 27%. Cancer studies are generally less conclusive, however, due in part to varying etiologies of cancers across sites.

In 2012, the German Nutrition Society[2] evaluated the evidence on vegetable and fruit consumption and found that increasing consumption was "convincing" for reducing hypertension, CHD, and stroke; "probable" for cancers; and "possible" for weight gain, as well as cognitive performance and Alzheimer's. Conversely, there was "probable" evidence for no association with T2DM independent of obesity, which is the strongest risk factor. The study also found that fruit and vegetables were possibly protective for chronic obstructive pulmonary disease, asthma, and rheumatoid arthritis; additional studies since 2012 have also shown a protective association with arthritis. There was insufficient evidence in connection with glaucoma and diabetic retinopathy. Note, however, that the more specific the disease and its mechanism and the fewer people affected—which limit a study's power as well as the total number of studies performed available for reviewing—the more difficult detecting dietary effects becomes. Therefore, as there are many animal and laboratory studies showing protective associations and bioactivity with phytonutrients, there is reason to believe that stronger conclusions may be revealed in human studies (of diseases like inflammatory bowel disease and eye disease) as science advances. Further, certain diseases are more likely to be affected by produce subgroups due to particular phytochemicals, which is why examining individual vegetables and fruits remains important.

While effects vary in magnitude, with the strongest associations shown in the prevention of heart disease and stroke, the 2015 Scientific Report from the Dietary Guidelines for Americans Advisory Committee concluded that "[v]egetables and fruit are the only characteristics of the diet that were consistently identified in every conclusion statement across health outcomes." Still, most Americans do not come close to the amount recommended to reduce preventable chronic diseases. The World Health Organization (WHO) reported that approximately 5.2 million deaths worldwide were attributable to inadequate vegetable and fruit consumption in 2013 and suggests eating *at least* 400 g daily as part of a healthy diet to promote health and prevent chronic diseases.

Finally, the low energy density of produce due to its high water and fiber content makes it a logical target in obesity studies. And advice from professional organizations and health advocates abounds to encourage consumption to manage weight or facilitate weight loss. Unfortunately, a subtle but important message is often missing: vegetables and fruit only facilitate weight loss if *replacing* higher-calorie foods. Simply adding a salad to every meal, even if nutrient-rich, will lead to weight gain if calories aren't otherwise in check; swapping berries for ice cream and veggies for cookies and chips (and the like) is necessary. Vegetables and fruits aren't magical weight loss tools, and study after study has shown that substitution is the key, not addition: weight loss will only come if the switch results in negative energy balance.

10

WHOLE GRAINS, REFINED GRAINS, AND GLUTEN

What are cereal grains and "pseudograins"?

Grains like wheat, corn, oats, and rice are cereal grasses, the fruit or seed of the grass family; many grains are thus referred to as "cereals." Some plants from the broadleaf family, like amaranth, buckwheat, and quinoa, are grouped with grains because they have a comparable macro- and micronutrient composition and are similarly consumed. (They are sometimes referred to as "pseudograins.") Grains are the richest source of carbohydrate in the diet and provide heart-healthy unsaturated fats, B-complex vitamins, minerals, fiber, and an array of phytochemicals that varies by plant. Grains are also the major protein source for many in the developing world. Without these cereal staples, many of which are below, billions would starve.

- **Amaranth:** particularly high in lysine (otherwise found largely in animal products), a good choice for vegans.
- **Barley:** rich in beta-glucans, a fiber shown to lower low-density lipoprotein ("bad") cholesterol (LDL); "pearled" barley has had some of the bran removed, while "hulled" has not.
- **Buckwheat:** aka, kasha (when toasted); botanically a seed, rich in rutin, a flavonoid; gluten-free.
- **Corn:** dried kernels are grains (like popcorn), while fresh corn is considered a vegetable; gluten-free.
- **Millet:** comes in white, gray, yellow, or red; high in copper.

- **Oat:** steel-cut and whole rolled are comparable in nutrition, though "quick-cooking" often has some fiber removed (to hasten preparation); associated with lower LDL; gluten-free.
- **Quinoa:** botanically a seed that comes in red, white, and black; almost twice the protein of other grains and includes all of the essential amino acids and many micronutrients; gluten-free.
- **Rice:** black, brown, and red are common colors; high in manganese; gluten-free.
- **Rye:** robust flavor with similar nutrition to barley and wheat; mainly used in the US to make whiskey.
- **Sorghum:** aka, guinea corn, dura, milo; rich in anthocyanins; gluten-free.
- **Wheat:** aka, bulgur, spelt, emmer, einkorn, durum, farro, cracked wheat, and wheat berries; white winter wheat and summer red wheat are common varieties: the former is softer and milder and used in "white whole wheat flour," whereas the latter gives (regular) whole wheat flour its red–brown hue.
- **Wild rice:** botanically a grass; provides iron and protein; gluten-free.

Rice, wheat, and maize comprise 60% of the world's energy intake in today's diets, whether consumed intact or through flours used in a vast array of foods the world over, bread to pasta, tortillas to tamales, cookies to crackers.

What's the difference between "whole" and "refined" grains?

All grains have a hull (hard outer shell), which is inedible and always removed before consumption. Whether a grain is "whole" or "refined" refers to how it's further processed before getting to eaters. A "whole grain" includes three major parts of the plant: bran (outer fibrous layer), germ (reproductive organ, rich in polyunsaturated fats, vitamins, and minerals), and endosperm (starchy interior that provides energy). For millennia, whole grains were consumed in porridges, breads, and other dietary staples. All of this changed during the Industrial Revolution, which brought mechanization to feed a growing population. An automated milling process removed the bran and germ, leaving only the sweeter, whiter endosperm, now referred to as a "refined" grain.

Refined grains are easier and quicker to cook and more shelf-stable as the oil-containing germ, which can become rancid, has been removed. Americans and western Europeans began to prefer the milder flavor of foods made with refined grains, like white bread, compared to their heartier counterparts with their darker colors and toothsome textures. There are sociological reasons, too, rooted in race, class, culture, and xenophobia: the color difference came to reflect a "refined" palate associated with higher wealth and incomes—and those individuals usually had white skin.

Refining grains also reduces many valuable nutrients. For example, vitamins B_1, B_2, B_3, B_6, E, K, and folate; minerals magnesium, potassium, iron, calcium, and selenium; and fiber and protein are all lower in white flour compared to whole wheat flour. To address this issue, some nutrients are added back to the refined grain mixture through "enrichment," namely thiamin, riboflavin, niacin, folate, and iron. Fiber is not added back, however, which is a significant loss in diet quality as most people don't consume enough for good health. Thus, while calories are similar—micronutrients and fiber have negligible energy content—whole grains are more nutrient-dense.

What is gluten, and are gluten-free diets important for health?

Gluten is an insoluble protein found in several cereal grasses, notably wheat, barley, and rye. Its physiochemical properties provide desirable baking qualities, like elasticity, structure, and volume, which is why gluten-containing flours are favored for breads and pastries. Like other proteins, an allergic response to gluten can arise in some people. Celiac disease occurs when an immune reaction in the small intestine leads to atrophy and malabsorption. (Wheat allergy is a separate disease with its own mechanism.) While screening and diagnosis of celiac disease have improved and underdiagnosis is still an issue, the prevalence has increased from 0.03% in the 1970s to about 1% (0.5–1.26%) in 2017 in both Europe and the US. Algerians have the highest prevalence (5.6%) and Japanese and Chinese the lowest. Gluten-related disorders have also increased, including non-celiac gluten sensitivity (NCGS) and gluten intolerances, estimated at about 6% in the US; NCGS presents with numerous gastrointestinal symptoms but is not an autoimmune disease.

Dietary, environmental, and genetic differences contribute to gluten disorders (such as in the varying frequency of *HLA-DG2* and other genetic variants), though the precise reasons for the rapid increase in celiac and other gluten disorders remain unclear. Consumption of wheat and vital gluten (which is separated from the starch component of wheat to impart desirable food processing properties) has increased globally, and some studies suggest that the timing of introduction of gluten and wheat into the diet during infancy and breastfeeding may play a role. Others have questioned whether changes in wheat production enhancing gluten content might be a factor, although agricultural data from the past century do not support this hypothesis. More recently, fermentable oligo-, di-, and monosaccharides and polyols (commonly known as "FODMAPS"), a group of sugars found in grains as well as some vegetables and fruits, have been associated with gastrointestinal distress. Research is currently investigating their potential roles in gluten-related disorders as the two are highly correlated.

Interest in gluten-free (GF) diets has climbed substantially in the past decade, due in part to increased prevalence, media attention, and the common occurrence of gastrointestinal issues. But gluten misinformation, demonization, and celebrity nutrition (GF is the most popular Hollywood diet) also play a role. Indeed, recent polls indicate around 25% (!) of American adults are going gluten-free, particularly women aged 20–39. The market for GF foods is booming, estimated at an annual growth rate of 10.4%. Yet there is no reason those without diagnosed gluten-related conditions should cut gluten-containing foods from their diet. There is no evidence to show that GF diets are helpful for weight loss—beyond any independent effect due to calorie deficit—or beneficial for heart disease prevention. While GF foodstuffs have improved considerably in taste and texture, many remain higher in sugar, sodium, and saturated fat and lower in fiber, B-complex vitamins, minerals, and phytonutrients compared to their whole grain counterparts. Thus, a number of studies have even found that those consuming GF diets have a poorer overall diet because vital nutrients can be compromised without careful dietary planning, as can happen whenever entire food groups are removed from the diet.

Do whole and refined grains differently impact the body?

While many strive to cut gluten, hence grains, from their diets under the pretense of better health, scientific research continues to accumulate showing that diets rich in whole grains are beneficial for gastrointestinal health and beyond. Studies including randomized controlled trials (RCTs) have shown that consuming whole grains leads to a significant reduction in LDL and that oats are particularly effective. A 2017 study including 21 meta-analyses observed 18% and 11% reductions in cardiovascular disease (CVD) and cancer mortality, respectively, among those consuming approximately 2–3 servings (45 g) of whole grains daily; protective effects for type 2 diabetes, cardiovascular disease (CVD), and colorectal, pancreatic, and gastric cancers were also observed. Stronger effects were obtained for a 90-g intake, with risk reductions occurring through 7–7½ servings daily for many health outcomes; whole grain bread, whole grain breakfast cereals, and added bran, as well as total bread and total breakfast cereals, were independently associated with reduced risks of CVD and all-cause mortality. An additional meta-analysis of 20 studies showed 25% and 6% lower risks of mortality from CVD and cancer, respectively, for each additional 3 servings (90 g) of whole grains.

Whole grain benefits are likely due not to any single component or biological mechanism but, rather, to their additive and synergistic effects in the body. Newer studies are showing beneficial results of whole grains on the microbiome, a function of their prebiotic fibers and resistant starches that feed "good" bacteria (Chapter 4). And a greater variety of whole grains led to both a higher amount and a greater diversity of gut microbes. There may also be undiscovered phytochemicals that contribute.

Many observational studies also show that whole grains have small but favorable effects on body weight, a function of their metabolic effects on appetite, satiety, nutrient availability, and energy utilization. Evidence from RCTs isolating a specific effect of whole grains on weight loss has been inconsistent, however.[1] Type and amount of grains consumed may play a role, as well as the nature of consumption (e.g., hot or cold, which impacts glycemic index).

One might expect refined grains to have a deleterious effect on health, given their higher glycemic index and lower nutrient content compared to whole grains. Interestingly, the extant literature is equivocal, though swapping whole grains for refined grains appears beneficial among diabetics. Isolating the effects of singular elements, even a food group, is challenging due to correlations with other dietary and behavioral elements. There are likely genetic and other biological factors involved, too, that impact metabolic processes. Several intriguing studies recently showed that white sourdough bread, which contains live bacteria and yeast, did not lead to expected changes in glucose and insulin in some people—and neither did non-sourdough white bread. The authors hypothesized differential effects on the microbiome (Chapter 4) and other factors may have impacted glycemic response. The studies were small and findings need to be reproduced, but underscore the phenomenon that the same foods can have different effects on different people, another harbinger of personalized nutrition (Chapter 18).

Insulin sensitivity is also directly related to body mass index (BMI). Thus, those with a healthy body weight are better able to manage the sugar boost from refined grains. And impact on blood sugar is related to what else is consumed in the meal alongside refined grains. Even though refined grains on their own don't always show a negative impact on health, studies of total dietary patterns that consider all intakes in concert show that consumers with higher intakes of refined grain foods—like cookies, crackers, pizza, white bread, pasta, and rice—do have a higher BMI, more T2DM, and greater risk of CVD. Here, and elsewhere, the total composition of the diet is more important than any individual food or food group.

How do you ensure grains are "whole"?

It takes a bit of effort to figure out which grains are "whole," due to crowded food packaging with misleading labels. To ensure the healthier option:

- **Look** for the word "whole" on the ingredient list (e.g., whole oats, whole wheat, whole corn); "enriched" does not mean whole, nor does "fortified."
- **Ignore** the food color, which is often adjusted to a browner hue to appear healthier.
- **Understand** that "multigrain" simply means that more than one grain is included: a multigrain bread may have wheat, corn, and oats, for example, but unless it's made with *whole wheat*, *whole corn*, and *whole oats*, it's not whole grain—even if it has added bran, fiber, or seeds.
- **Check** the supermarket bulk bins for whole grains, where they are lower in price and have less packaging.
- **Remember** basic nutrition principles: processed foods such as granola bars may be "100% whole grain" since they're made with whole oats—but are often loaded in added sugar, sodium, and calories.

11

PLANT PROTEIN POWER

BEANS AND PEAS, LEGUMES AND PULSES, NUTS AND SEEDS

What are legumes, and why are they unique in nutrition and agriculture?

A legume is the fruit or seed of plants including beans (e.g., black, kidney, pinto, lima, fava, soy), peas (e.g., split, green, black-eyed), and lentils. There are about 20 legume species currently consumed by humans. Protein is 20–25% by weight, around 2–3 times the amount found in cereals and on par with many animal foods. Legumes are low in total fat and rich in iron, zinc, potassium, magnesium, phosphorus, B-complex vitamins, fiber, and phytonutrients like phytosterols and phenolic acids. There are nutritional differences in species—kidney beans provide molybdenum, while lentils are particularly high in resistant starch—and their fiber and protein are satiating and provide sustained energy due to their low glycemic impact. Keeping no-sodium cans or frozen on hand or scooping dried from the supermarket's bulk bins is a convenient way to add a protein, fiber, and phytonutrient boost to meals.

Pulses are a subgroup of legumes that produce edible seeds, which are then harvested as dry grains. Some additional plants are also leguminous, like clover, alfalfa, lupins, and peanuts. Despite these botanical definitions, nutritionists often group foods according to nutrient composition and/or consumption pattern (as with whole grains and pseudograins, Chapter 10). This is why peanuts, which are much higher in fat than other legumes, are grouped with nuts and seeds. Similarly, although green peas are technically legumes, they count as vegetables when consumed fresh—and are considered pulses if consumed dried. (Whoa; this is arguably beyond what everyone needs to know.)

Legumes are unique among plants because, through a chemical reaction with certain bacteria (e.g., *Rhizobium, Bradyrhizobium*), atmospheric nitrogen is converted into a form of nitrogen used to nourish plants and fertilize the soil. Some legumes can also free phosphorus in soil. Legumes are often used in crop rotation and intercropping in eco-conscious farming for these reasons. They also have broad genetic diversity and, hence, are well poised to enable selection and breeding of climate-resilient varieties. Compared to animal foods, legumes require fewer resources like water, land, and fuel to produce per calorie; are less expensive; have a longer shelf life; and are a major crop and protein source among subsistence and smallholder farmers in the developing world. Pulses are so critical to human and environmental health and global food security that the Food and Agriculture Organization of the United Nations (FAO) deemed 2016 the "International Year of Pulses."

How do legumes impact weight and health?

Legumes' unique nutritional profile is beneficial in myriad physiological activities. For instance, the fermentation of insoluble fibers in the large bowel produces short-chain fatty acids, which provide energy to colonocytes (i.e., colon cells) and may inhibit tumor formation. Fiber-containing foods like legumes also contain phenolic antioxidants, thought to play a role in cancer due to their beneficial gastrointestinal effects. A 2017 review of 111 prospective cohort studies found no effect between legume consumption and colorectal cancer, however.

Yet evidence is strong that consuming 130 grams per day (about 1 serving) of pulses significantly lowers low-density lipoprotein ("bad") cholesterol (LDL). A similar dose of pulses (132 g/d) was associated with greater weight loss compared to other diets with the same number of calories and was helpful in weight maintenance in an analysis of 21 randomized controlled trials (RCTs). Reviews based on a smaller number of observational studies and RCTs indicated that legumes are also associated with an approximate 10% lower risk of both cardiovascular disease and coronary heart disease; no significant reductions in stroke or T2DM were observed.

Researchers emphasize the need for studies with more participants and longer follow-up. They point out that results may reflect intrinsic properties of legumes, substitution effects from replacing less healthy protein sources, or the aggregate role of legumes as part of an overall dietary pattern.

While most investigations in humans examine total legume consumption, there are differences among types, like variability in fibers, oligosaccharides, polysaccharides, proteins, and phytochemicals, that require individual study, like soy. Yet other studies consider total dietary patterns, finding that those high in legumes are particularly healthful, like the Mediterranean and Okinawan diets (Chapter 17). Studies like these that consider the whole diet are vital as "[t]he synergistic or antagonistic effects of these phytochemical mixtures from food legumes, their interaction with other components of the diet, and the mechanism of their action" are key to understanding their protective role.

Why do beans produce gas (and can it be mitigated)?

Humans produce 1–4 pints of gas daily, comprising nitrogen, hydrogen, carbon dioxide, oxygen, and, in some, methane. (Sulfur may also be present following consumption of foods like cruciferous vegetables.) Gas is excreted through either the mouth or anus 13–21 times daily. There are various factors that contribute to gas, including dietary factors like legumes.

Beans' insoluble fiber contributes to gas. Beans also contain the indigestible oligosaccharides stachyose, verbascose, and raffinose. These sugars pass through the gastrointestinal tract and are fermented by bacteria in the gut, creating gas. Gas may cause gastrointestinal discomfort before it is excreted through the anus. However, gas may be reabsorbed back into blood or consumed by intestinal bacteria.

Gas is a healthy metabolic byproduct of consuming foods with indigestible components. Indeed, some of beans' salubrious effects are a result of the fermentation process. Some research suggests that gradually increasing the amount of fiber in the diet can help reduce gaseous effects. Consuming alpha-galactosidase (a digestive enzyme produced from the fungus *Aspergillus niger*) can ameliorate the gas produced by the oligosaccharides, though it is contraindicated in certain health conditions. Over-the-counter remedies can reduce abdominal discomfort. Herbs such as anise, fennel, and peppermint purportedly aid in digestion, though research is lacking.

Why is soy unique, and how is it related to health?

Soybeans are distinct because they provide all of the essential amino acids; calcium, selenium, flavonoids, and phytosterols; isoflavones like genistein and daidzein; and phytoestrogens that interact with human estrogen by either mimicking or blocking its actions. Soybeans can be enjoyed fresh, dried, steamed (edamame), canned, or frozen. Soy is rich in polyunsaturated fats and provides about 300 calories, 68 g of protein, and 17 g of fiber per cup.

Soybeans have been used for millennia to create a wide variety of foodstuffs in the human diet. Ground soybeans cooked in water make soymilk; if a coagulant is added to the mixture, curds will arise and create tofu when pressed into cakes. Pressed beans create soybean oil, and the remainder can be dried and ground into flour. Soy protein concentrate, marketed as either texturized soy protein (aka, TSP) or texturized vegetable protein (aka, TVP), results from defatted soy flour that has been cooked under pressure, then either rehydrated or dried; one-half cup of dried TSP has 24 g of protein and 8 g of fiber. (Seitan—"wheat meat"—is often lumped in with soy protein products due to similarity in texture and use, though it's made from gluten.) Additional soy foods are made with beans that have undergone microbial fermentation using such things as bacteria, fungi, or molds. Water added to fermented crushed soybeans produces soy sauce; salt and fungus added to fermented soybeans yields miso, a thick paste; and tempeh is made from fermented whole soybeans, creating a chewier and firmer texture than tofu.

Soy has received copious research attention due to its unique nutritional composition and prominent role in the Japanese diet; the Okinawans are among the longest-lived, healthiest groups in the world. The evidence is very strong that soy lowers LDL and soy protein in particular may be effective; effects are similar in those with and without T2DM, although soy has no effect among those with familial hypercholesterolemia. (The latter finding is similar to other diet interventions, which can't always overcome genetic predisposition.) There is some evidence to show that soy may also lower triglycerides and improve blood sugar and insulin sensitivity, with a 2010 review showing that fermented soy foods were particularly effective. No studies have shown a direct effect between soy consumption and lower risk of heart disease or T2DM.

Soy was hypothesized to be protective in relation to hormone-related conditions (like hot flashes) and diseases like breast cancer, due to its phytoestrogens, though early evidence showed both protective and harmful effects. A 2013 meta-analysis of 131 studies comparing soy to placebo, including 40 RCTs and 80 observational studies, found no reductions in hot flashes; null relations between soy and breast cancer incidence or recurrence, including among women taking tamoxifen (a drug used in the secondary prevention of breast cancer); and no increase in circulating estradiol or impacts on estrogen-responsive target tissues. However, higher soy consumption consistent with traditional Japanese diets—2–3 servings daily including 25–50 isoflavones—may reduce breast cancer risk. Interestingly, some studies show beneficial effects of soy only in Asian women. Life course epidemiology suggests that timing matters: soy may be protective if consumed early in life, perhaps "learning" to interact with the body's hormones to restructure the risk of disease during growth and development. Genetics certainly also plays a role.

Soy science continues to evolve, with some studies showing protective effects on endometrial and prostate cancers and bone health, though stronger data are needed. Newer studies suggest that eating soy as a whole food may have different effects from consuming only its protein or just its isoflavones in high-dose supplements. And soy's role in health may be due not only to its diverse properties but because it supplants less nutritious animal-based protein foods from the diet. Likewise, soy may be just one component of a dietary pattern beneficial for heart disease and cancer reduction. The 2015–2020 Dietary Guidelines for Americans thus continues to recommend soy foods of all kinds for health and disease prevention (up to 8½ ounce equivalents weekly).

What's in a nut?

A true nut, like a chestnut, is the fruit of a plant that grows on a tree, its outermost layer (ovary wall) becoming a hard shell upon maturity. Nut and seed botany becomes quite complex, and nutrition and culinary classification are more useful for everyday eaters. "Tree nuts" include almond, Brazil, cashew, hazelnut, macadamia, pecan, pine, pistachio, and walnut. The "groundnut" peanut (aka, goober) is a legume whose fruit ripens underground within a pod. All nuts are fruits (ripened ovaries) of a plant, while seeds are the ripened and fertilized ovule. Nuts and seeds can be consumed raw following some processing—almond skins naturally contain cyanide, for instance—but toasting or roasting enhances flavor and crunch.

Nuts and seeds are nutrient-rich but also energy-dense due to their high fat content, composing 50% or more of their weight. A small handful packs 160–200 calories per ounce, while smaller seeds (like chia, flax, sesame) have 130–160 calories per 2 tablespoons. Both contain some saturated fat but are known for their heart-healthy mixture of polyunsaturated (PUFA) and monounsaturated fatty acids (MUFA). Nuts and seeds also include protein, vitamin E, fiber, zinc, calcium, magnesium, potassium, selenium, and phosphorus and various phytochemicals (e.g., flavonoids, lignans, phenols, resveratrol, lutein). They are a particularly important source of protein and nutrients in the developing world.

Phytochemical and micronutrient concentrations vary by nut: almonds are known for vitamin E, Brazil nuts (grown only in the Amazon) for selenium, peanuts for polyphenols (particularly resveratrol), pecans for most total carotenoids, and walnuts for highest antioxidant concentration. Chia and flax seeds are protein powerhouses, with 11 and 8 g in 2 tablespoons, respectively, while sesame and hemp include all of the essential amino acids. Walnuts, flax, chia, and hemp contain omega-3 essential fatty acids; hemp also has omega-6. Pressing nuts and seeds extracts their oils, which then have about 110 calories per tablespoon (9 calories per gram)—and removes much of the other nutrition found in the whole plant excepting fat-soluble components like vitamin E. Nuts are also an important source of protein and nutrients, particularly in the developing world.

Are nuts fattening, or associated with increased risk of disease?

Like many high-fat foods, nuts and seeds were vilified in the 1980s—and many people still rely on this outdated science to guide food choices. Yet both can be part of a healthy diet when consumed in moderation as part of an energy-balanced diet. Indeed, the protein and fat together contribute to satiety (i.e., a feeling of fullness), which can help reduce calorie intake. There are additional properties of nuts that are conducive to a healthy weight, including increased thermogenesis (an aspect of energy expenditure) and fat oxidation.

Observational data, including prospective studies, have shown that those consuming up to 4 servings of nuts weekly do not have a different body weight from nonconsumers—in other words, a diet including nuts does not lead to overweight—while others suggest that a small handful of nuts daily may even result in lower body mass index (BMI) and body weight compared to nonconsumers. (Seeds are less commonly consumed so are often grouped with nuts in epidemiologic studies.) Effects may be in part due to their role in aggregate, as nuts are often consumed as part of a healthful Mediterranean diet pattern, or because they replace less nutritious snacks like chips and cookies. In any case, findings from 33 RCTs are consistent with observational studies, showing that participants who include nuts of various kinds do not have a higher body weight, BMI, or waist circumference compared to those on a control diet, including those following a "low-fat" regimen.

There is strong evidence from 61 RCTs indicating that nuts are associated with lower LDL and blood pressure. Countless studies have also shown associations between nuts and a lower risk of coronary artery disease and hypertension as well as coronary heart disease and cardiovascular mortality. Most available data do not show a significant relation with stroke or T2DM, and there are limited reports on nuts and cancer. Newer hypotheses regarding the role of nuts on cognition and brain health, including synergistic effects with berries, are now being tested.

What's the current science on nut allergies and prevention?

The global prevalence of food allergies has risen in the past several decades—and doubled in some Western countries—and both tree nuts and peanuts may cause reactions. Nut allergies are among the most common, particularly that to peanuts. Allergies to one tree nut often translate to other species due to protein similarities. A 2015 review of 36 studies around the world estimated the prevalence of nut allergies at around 2%, ranging from 0.05% to 4.9%. Peanut allergy can be fatal in extreme cases.

As with many serious food-related health conditions, abstinence is often the first line of defense when data are sparse, and many mothers were initially instructed to avoid nuts completely during pregnancy and nursing, as well as with young children, to curtail development of allergies. Yet many studies have since shown that restricting nuts has the opposite effect: women completely avoiding nuts in effect oversensitized their offspring, who were in turn more likely to develop allergies. One striking RCT among 640 high-risk infants suffering from known egg allergy and eczema, the Learning Early About Peanut Allergy (LEAP) study, found that the group consuming peanuts had a far lower prevalence of peanut allergies at age 5 compared to those avoiding peanuts completely. This study and others suggest that early exposure to potential allergens increases healthy immune responses that decrease the likelihood of developing food allergies.

As a result of the landmark LEAP study and other data, many health organizations revised their earlier recommendations to parents, including the National Institute of Allergy and Infectious Diseases in January 2017. Today when to provide allergen-containing foods and in what amounts to kids with differing risk levels are now provided to reduce the probability of developing a peanut allergy.

12

LAND ANIMALS AND
ANIMAL-BASED FOODS

What animals are consumed for food, and how do they
differ nutritionally?

Between 1970 and 2011, the number of animals raised for food
increased three-fold, from 7.3 billion to 24.2 billion. A wide variety
of animals are eaten across the world and contribute up to one-third
of global protein consumption and 15% of calories. One billion of the
world's poorest in South Asia and sub-Saharan Africa depend on
livestock for food and livelihoods. Domesticated animals like cattle,
pigs, and poultry as well as buffalo, sheep (lamb), and goats are
most commonly consumed. Camel, yak, crocodile, kangaroo, horse,
snake, ostrich, wild game, dog, and bushmeat may also be found
on some tables. Entomophagy (eating insects) is practiced by more
than 2 billion worldwide, and a majority of the 1900 edible species
are enjoyed around the world, mainly in Africa and Asia, often as
delicacy (not as necessity). The four most commonly consumed
species are in the orders Coleoptera (beetle; 31%), Lepidoptera (cat-
erpillar, butterfly, moth; 18%), Hymenoptera (bee, wasp, ant; 14%),
and Orthoptera (grasshopper, cricket; 13%).

More pork is eaten globally than any other meat, comprising 36%
of total animal intake, followed by poultry (35%) and beef (22%).
Goats are common in many places in the developing world as they
are more easily raised than many animals, can live in diverse climates,
and produce milk. Goats are also favored throughout the Caribbean,
Southeast Asia, and Africa. While goat doesn't surpass pork in total
consumption, it is the most widely consumed animal: about 75% of

the world's population eats goat. Though it remains rare on Western tables, goat's attractiveness is growing as a highly nutritious—and more sustainable—alternative to beef.

Animal foods are a big part of both American and British diets. In the US, increased production per capita is expected for beef (6.1%), pork (5.4%), and chicken (2.1%). These estimates from the US Department of Agriculture (USDA) reflect supply-side numbers and are a result, in part, of low feed grain prices. While the numbers overestimate consumption, as some food is wasted, they are nonetheless proxies for domestic dining habits once imports and exports are considered. In particular, 222.2 pounds (100.8 kg) of red meat and poultry will be available to consume per person on average in 2018—more than 100 billion pounds in total—reaching an all-time high since these data were first measured in 1970. (The market for plant-based meat products, in contrast, is expected to be around $750 million in 2018.) Much of the growth is driven by poultry, which has been rising since 1990 as beef (including lamb, mutton, and veal) has been declining and pork has remained fairly stable. Indeed, chicken production has increased five-fold since 1970, while beef has remained largely unchanged. Still, beef consumption in the US is currently around four times the global average, topped only by Brazil, Argentina, and Uruguay.

Like plants, animals differ somewhat in their nutritional composition, although protein and several micronutrients are the main players. The key nutrients beyond protein found in commonly consumed animals in Western diets follow.

- **Cow:** zinc, iron, selenium, phosphorus, vitamin B_{12}, vitamin B_6, riboflavin, niacin, vitamin B_5, saturated fat, monounsaturated fat, cholesterol
- **Pig:** thiamin, niacin, vitamin B_6, vitamin B_{12}, selenium, phosphorus, zinc, iron
- **Chicken:** selenium, phosphorus, niacin, vitamin B_6, monounsaturated fat, saturated fat (skin only)
- **Turkey:** niacin, vitamin B_6, riboflavin, potassium, selenium, phosphorus, zinc, iron, saturated fat (skin only)
- **Goat:** vitamin B_{12}, iron, potassium, zinc, cholesterol
- **Lamb:** vitamin B_{12}, selenium, vitamin B_6, zinc, phosphorus, monounsaturated fat, saturated fat, cholesterol

- **Buffalo:** vitamin B$_{12}$, vitamin B$_6$, potassium, iron, zinc, copper, selenium

While animal flesh has comparable protein, differing fat composition drives variation in calorie content (Table 12.1). Of note, the iron in animal foods, called heme iron, is more readily absorbed (bioavailable) in humans compared to non-heme iron, the kind found in plants. Red meat includes beef, veal, pork, lamb, mutton, horse, and goat. Processed meat is modified in some way to become more shelf-stable and tasty, often through the addition of salt and other additives. Red and processed meats (RPM) have received much research attention over the years due to their prominence in Western diets. They are an established risk factor for colorectal cancer (Chapter 4). Many studies have also shown significant associations between RPM and type 2 diabetes mellitus (T2DM) and heart disease, particularly for processed meat. A 2017 study showed a 37% increased risk in heart disease for each daily intake of 50 g of processed meat among those with T2DM, while a 17% increase was seen for a 100-g daily intake of red meat. An enormous study in Europe also showed an 18% increase in all-cause mortality per 50-g daily intake of processed meat, driven mainly by cardiovascular diseases (CVD). A later study confirmed these findings and showed an association with red meat, although findings were only apparent in Americans; intakes were not high enough in European or Asian populations to detect an effect, perhaps.

Table 12.1 Nutrient Comparison of 5 Commonly Consumed Meats, Per 3-Ounce Portion, Roasted*

Meat	Calories	Protein (g)	Iron (g)	Saturated Fat (g)	Total Fat (g)
Beef	245	23	2.0	6.8	16.0
Chicken	120	21	1.5	1.1	3.5
Pork	310	21	2.7	8.7	24.0
Lamb	235	22	1.4	7.3	16.0
Goat	122	23	3.2	0.79	2.58

*Data are from the USDA National Nutrient Database for Standard Reference (Release 28, released September 2015, slightly revised May 2016).

Many animal foods contain conjugated linoleic acid (CLA), an essential fatty acid that can only be obtained through diet. Some refer to CLA as a "zoonutrient" since it is found primarily in animal foods, although a few plant foods provide minute amounts of CLA (e.g., sunflower and safflower oils). CLA is higher in grass-fed animals compared to those raised on grain. Some animal experiments and a few human studies suggest that high doses of CLA can increase fat-burning, reduce inflammation, and improve glucose metabolism. While often championed as a weight loss elixir, the evidence is limited that CLA has appreciable effects on either losing weight or building muscle.

What resources are needed for animal production?

Almost 30% of the planet's ice-free surface is dedicated to livestock grazing, which has degraded about 20% of the world's grasslands. Meat production requires large swaths of land and hence is the largest contributor to deforestation: approximately 13 billion hectares of forest are lost annually to agricultural use. The Food and Agriculture Organization of the United Nations (FAO) estimates that forests comprised 31.6% of the world's land in 1990 (4128 hectares) and 30.6% in 2015 (3999 hectares), with the largest losses in Africa and South America. Deforestation removes trees—a critical carbon "sink" that reduces atmospheric carbon dioxide (CO_2)—and cleared land is used as pasture for livestock or cropland for plants. Deforestation is the second leading source of atmospheric CO_2 (the most abundant greenhouse gas [GHG]), following fossil fuel combustion. Forests are essential for replenishing groundwater supplies that are vital for agriculture, drinking, and other industrial and human uses. They also protect soil and biodiversity: more than half of all terrestrial animals, plants, and insects live in forests.

Part of the land used in agriculture—about one-third of all cropland—is for growing animal feed. In the US, the main feed crop is corn (96.2%), followed by sorghum (2.5%), barley (1%), and oats (0.4%). In fact, the vast majority of corn is fed to animals; thus, the resources used in production—fuel, water, land, fertilizer—also contribute greatly to the environmental cost of raising animals for food. About 92% of freshwater on the planet is used for agriculture, and about one-third of this is associated with animal foods and products.

Mekonnen and Hoekstra compared the water footprint from various animals and plants using data from China, India, The Netherlands, and the US, finding that the average water footprint per calorie for beef is 20-fold higher than that for cereals and starchy roots. Similarly, the footprint per gram of protein for milk, eggs, and chicken was 1.5-fold larger than that for pulses. Comparing animal foods, the water footprint of beef was 15 415 m^3/ton, far higher than that for sheep/goat (8763 m^3/ton), pig (5988 m^3/ton), or poultry (4325 m^3/ton). Livestock production requires water for animal consumption as well as to irrigate feed crops and pasture. Conventional beef (versus grass-fed) is particularly intensive as the water required to grow feed crops dwarfs that needed for hydration and care (e.g., washing). Conversely, vegetables (322 m^3/ton), starchy roots (387 m^3/ton), fruits (962 m^3/ton), and cereals (1644 m^3/ton) were among the crops with the smallest water footprints.[1]

A 2014 report from the *Proceedings of the National Academy of Sciences* used life cycle assessment methods (a process that quantifies the various elements in agriculture) to calculate the land, irrigation water, GHGs, and reactive nitrogen (Nr, used in fertilizer) costs of beef, pork, poultry, hens (for eggs), and cows (for dairy production). Findings showed that beef utilized 28 times more land, 11 times more irrigation water, 5 times more GHGs, and 6 times more Nr on average compared to other livestock categories. When compared to potatoes, wheat, and rice, beef used 160 times more land, 8 times more irrigation water, 11 times more GHGs, and 19 times more Nr. Part of the reason for the major difference in resource use is that cows are three to six times less efficient at converting food to protein and calories ("feed conversion efficiency"), thus requiring more resources to obtain as many calories compared to other livestock. Cows are also ruminant animals that consume and digest cellulose (from grass) and expel the gas through a process called "enteric methanogenesis," which produces the majority of atmospheric methane. Methane is a GHG about 21 times more potent than CO_2. In fact, livestock-related GHGs contribute about two-thirds of all agricultural emissions, including manure left on pasture (16%) and manure management (7%), in addition to enteric fermentation (40%).

Some improvements have been made regarding livestock production. FAO estimated that net annual forest loss decreased from 0.18% to 0.08% between 1990 and 2015 due to improved management and conservation—with a resultant 25% reduction in carbon emissions. Further, technologic advances in nutrition and genetics and improved farm management have reduced the environmental impact of beef production since the 1970s, resulting in decreases of 19% feed, 12% water, and 33% land with a concomitant 16% decrease in the carbon footprint per unit of beef. Likewise, the carbon footprint per billion kilograms of milk produced in 2007 was 37% lower than that produced in 1944. That said, a number of these gains are a direct result of the increased use of concentrated animal feeding operations (CAFOs) and growth-enhancing technologies to increase productivity and reduce life span. Furthermore, the increased use of corn in animal feed, which requires extensive irrigation, has increased the water footprint of beef by 42% during that same time frame.

What is a concentrated animal feeding operation (CAFO), and why does it matter?

An animal feeding operation (AFO) is defined by EPA as "a facility where animals are kept confined and fed or maintained for 45 or more days per year, and crops, vegetation, or forage growth are not sustained over a normal growing period"; "concentrated", per the AFO, refers specifically to the type and number of animals and in what density they were raised. (The word "confined" is sometimes also used.) There is little debate that AFOs and CAFOs are efficient, low-cost ways to produce meat, milk, and eggs. Yet conditions in both operations are often inhumane, with considerable animal suffering due to crowding, inability to move, lack of ventilation, inadequate temperature controls, and stress; these factors contribute to unsanitary conditions and ill health. This necessitates the use of prophylactic antibiotics in feed. And conventional feeding systems, as with crops, have favored a few species to further maximize efficiency: FAO estimates that six breeds account for 90% of cattle and that 20% of breeds are at risk of extinction as a result.

In 1972, the Clean Water Act identified AFOs and CAFOs as sources of pollution due to discharging waste into the environment, including both solid waste (manure) and wastewater. The US Environmental Protection Agency (EPA) estimates that livestock produce three to twenty times more solid waste than *all* Americans, around 1.2–1.37 billion tons—and, unlike for humans, there are no treatment facilities. Manure is often applied to land as it's a natural fertilizer, but it is used in levels exceeding what is needed for soil health, providing too much nitrogen and phosphorus. Manure may also contain potential pathogens (like *Escherichia coli*) and antibiotic-resistant bacteria, both human health risks, as well as chemical residues, animal blood, and copper sulfate, used in bovine footbaths. Manure often leaches into groundwater, and pathogens and traces of antibiotics, vaccines, and hormones have been detected in drinking water alongside waterborne pathogens. The odor—a result of gases like ammonia, methane, nitrous oxide, and hydrogen sulfide released primarily by manure but also from other processes on meat and dairy farms—is overwhelming and may be a risk factor for childhood asthma and other respiratory illnesses among nearby residents; nearby property values also tend be lower, unsurprisingly.

Agriculture is considered one of the most dangerous occupations in the world. Farmworkers in AFOs and CAFOs have increased proximity and exposure to pathogens as well as noxious gases and organic dust and, thus, an enhanced risk of a wide variety of respiratory illnesses such as chronic bronchitis, organic dust toxic syndrome, and syndromes related to mucous membrane inflammation and asthma. Musculoskeletal injuries are common due to repetitive tasks, as are traumatic injuries from dangerous machines and tools. Farmers, ranchers, and agricultural managers were on the "Top Ten" list of most dangerous jobs in the US, with a fatal work injury rate of 22 per 100 000 full-time equivalent workers—compared to the all-worker rate of 3.4. Of the 4836 total fatal work injuries reported in 2015, 252 were in this same group, second only to drivers and truck drivers. Agriculture, forestry, fishing, and hunting (counted together by the Bureau of Labor Statistics) had the highest incidence rate of nonfatal occupational injuries and illnesses in the private sector in 2015: 5.7 per 100 workers, or 56 100 individuals. And despite the gains made in the meatpacking industry more than a century ago following Upton Sinclair's *The Jungle* (Chapter 1), meatpacking was still ranked as one of the most dangerous jobs in the US in 2005. Only minor improvements have been seen since then, and there is concern about industry's underreporting of accidents, illnesses, and fatalities. Furthermore, these jobs remain mostly held by immigrants and people of color, who often suffer from exploitation, low wages, unsafe working conditions, and a lack of health insurance and job security.

For all of these reasons and more, there is widespread scientific consensus that meat production (including beef, poultry, and pork) is contributing to climate change as well as a host of other critical social, environmental, and health issues, many of which are exacerbated by CAFOs. In response, the US beef industry is currently analyzing the environmental impacts—though not the other critical issues—of representative feeding operations, considering "cradle-to-farm gate" footprints for greenhouse gas emission (GHGe), fossil-based fuel use, water use, and Nr loss. Still, meat consumption is rising in low- and middle-income countries due to increasing income and urbanization, particularly red and processed meat in China and Brazil. FAO estimates that demand will increase 74% for meat, 58% for dairy, and 500% for eggs by 2050. The problems faced by both planet and people will surely amplify if current production practices do not become more sustainable, healthful, and just.

Why are antibiotics used in CAFOs, and is it important for human health?

The World Health Organization (WHO) estimates that the majority of antibiotics are used in animal production—as much as 80% in some countries. Their main use is not as therapeutic treatment, however, but as antibiotic growth promoters that stimulate growth and, hence, reduce production costs. They are also used to prevent the spread of disease in crowded and unsanitary conditions of intensive feeding operations. In the US, antibiotics are used primarily in cows, chickens, and pigs.

The use of antibiotics in the livestock industry began in the middle of the 20th century and may be indicated in limited situations. Yet the evidence is clear that the overuse of antibiotics in animal production is at the root of antibiotic resistance, which is both an animal and a human health issue. That's because the antibiotics used in animal husbandry are the same as those used in humans. Due to overuse, the "bad" bacteria that antibiotics are designed to wipe out in animals become resistant, reproduce, and multiply, creating dangerous "superbugs." These antibiotic-resistant bacteria can then be transmitted to people either directly through meat consumption or indirectly through environmental contamination from animal excrement or infected land and water.

Scientists have concluded that the prolific overuse of antibiotics in animals is contributing greatly to antibiotic resistance in humans. Antibiotics commonly used in human medicine are therefore ineffective, increasing the risk of serious illness, disease, and death. As a result, many organizations around the world have called for the termination of antibiotic use for growth and prevention purposes in animals, as was done in Sweden in 1986 and throughout the European Union (EU) in 2006. In 2010, the US Food and Drug Administration (FDA) and acknowledged the association between antibiotics in meat production and antibiotic resistance in humans, and the Centers for Disease Control and Prevention (CDC) concluded that antibiotic resistance in human health was a *direct* result of antibiotic overuse in CAFOs.

The taste for meat and animal products is driving an increase in the use of antibiotics worldwide, particularly as countries like China are following farming practices used in the US. This is fueling the further spread of antibiotic resistance. According to Director-General of the WHO Dr. Tedros Adhanom Ghebreyesus, "[a] lack of effective antibiotics is as serious a security threat as a sudden and deadly disease outbreak." Fortunately, alternatives exist, including reducing confinement, utilizing vaccines, and improving hygiene. Indeed, a 2017 review of 181 studies found that interventions that restricted or banned antibiotic use, like organic farming, lowered antibiotic-resistant bacteria in animals by as much as 39%. And antibiotic resistance in humans was thus decreased by as much as 24%. The study led WHO to implement new guidelines for the use of antibiotics in agriculture, recommending that "farmers and the food industry stop using antibiotics routinely to promote growth and prevent disease in healthy animals" and that, when necessary, antibiotics should be selected from those deemed "least important" to human health rather than those of "highest priority / critically important." In the US, FDA asked the meat industry to stop using antibiotics as growth promoters in 2017 but did not address their use in prevention, thus allowing wide-scale use to continue. (Some companies are stepping up even so: in 2017, 15 major outlets agreed not to serve poultry raised with antibiotics, including McDonald's and KFC.)

Animal foods produced with antibiotics continue to confer a heightened health risk to farmworkers who raise them and eaters who consume them, as well as to the public health. A sobering UK report estimated that unless universal action is undertaken, which is necessary due to trade that moves superbugs across the globe, antibiotic resistance will kill 10 million people in 2050 alone, a considerable jump from the approximately 700 000 lives it currently takes annually (with an $8 trillion price tag in healthcare costs).

Why are hormones used in animal production?

FDA has approved the use of natural steroid hormones (e.g., estrogen, progesterone, testosterone) and their synthetic counterparts in animal production since 1950. Like antibiotics, these drugs enhance the growth rate and efficiency with which animals convert feed into meat and milk. Unlike antibiotics, steroid hormones are only used in cattle and sheep, not chickens or pigs; labels on poultry and pork stating "hormone-free" are nothing more than marketing gimmicks to garner sales.

One hormone commonly used in dairy cattle is recombinant bovine somatotropin (rBST; aka, bovine growth hormone, rBGH), which is used to stimulate milk production. Milk and dairy products from these cows have been on the market since 1993. FDA and others concluded initially and in a follow-up report from 2013 that milk from rBST-treated cows is as safe to drink as that from nontreated cows as its proteins do not differ from those produced naturally; residues, if present, have been deemed innocuous. (Animals fully metabolize these hormones before slaughter, virtually eliminating the probability of the steroids getting to humans.) Thus, although producers are permitted to label products as being free from rBST/rBGH, they are also legally obligated to include a statement that such milk has not been found to be any different from that of nontreated cows. Even so, the American Public Health Association and others oppose the use of hormones in dairy cattle—and the EU does not permit the use of hormones in any cattle.

The use of rBST for constant milk production can lead to increased pain and suffering. Not only is this behavior cruel, but it can result in infections like mastitis, which in turn leads to an increased use of antibiotics, thus creating a cycle dangerous to both cows and humans. For these reasons and others, the Humane Society of the US and the Humane Farming Association also oppose the use of rBST in dairy cows.

Who drinks milk, and what does it offer nutritionally?

Human infants produce the enzyme lactase, which metabolizes the lactose in breast milk. Yet most humans stop producing lactase early in life and thus become "lactose-intolerant," resulting in gastrointestinal discomfort due to the inability to properly digest and absorb milk and its products. Scientists estimate that 75% of humans globally are lactose-intolerant, which differs by ethnic background and geographic location. In the US, approximately 90% of Asian Americans, 74% of Native Americans, 70% of African Americans, and 53% of Mexican Americans are lactose-intolerant. Those with European ancestry are more likely to produce lactase throughout life, perhaps a result of a genetic mutation during human evolution.

Even so, many people throughout the world enjoy drinking milk, whether from cow, goat, camel, reindeer, llama, sheep, or water buffalo. FAO estimates that around 6 billion people worldwide consume milk and dairy products, mostly in the developing world. The highest milk consumption per capita is in Europe, Finland and Sweden in particular. Milk is nutrient-rich, an excellent source of protein, notably casein and whey. Milk also includes vitamins (e.g., riboflavin, vitamin B_{12}, pantothenic acid, vitamins A and D) and minerals (e.g., calcium, iodine, selenium, magnesium, phosphorus, zinc, potassium). The richness of whole milk comes from its fat (mostly saturated, some monounsaturated, scant polyunsaturated). The fat is partially removed in low-fat milks and fully removed in nonfat (skim) milk; this also removes its fat-soluble vitamins like A and D, which are often added back through fortification. If the milk comes from grass-fed animals, you'll get a few plant-based omega-3 fatty acids along with conjugated linoleic acid (CLA).

Animal milk is an important source of nutrients for children in the developing world in particular, where nutritious food is less plentiful; a goat, cow, or water buffalo on the family farm in India, Africa, or Asia provides essential nutrition that may be otherwise difficult to obtain. Conversely, drinking milk in the developed world is far from necessary given the many other food sources available to meet nutrient needs—not to mention the public health, animal welfare, environmental, and ethical considerations of raising animals discussed herein.

Are milk and its nutrients related to bone health and osteoporosis?

While plant-based foods (e.g., dark leafy greens, beans, tofu) and dietary supplements are good sources of calcium, milk and dairy are the main contributors if consumed. A 2014 study estimated that 10.2 million American adults aged 50 and above, around 1 in 10, had osteoporosis; by age 65, 5.1% of men and 24.5% of women had the disease. Globally, osteoporosis causes more than 8.9 million fractures annually and impacts 75 million people in Japan, Europe, and the US. The International Osteoporosis Foundation estimates that osteoporosis is responsible for more disability than noncommunicable diseases like asthma, rheumatoid arthritis, hypertension, and heart disease.

Osteoporosis has a strong genetic basis, like many diseases, but lifestyle factors such as diet also play a role. Both osteoporosis and low bone mass are conditions of aging: all adults begin losing bone mass starting as early as 30 years old, so building the strongest bones possible before then, particularly during early growth and development, is critical. Slowing the rate of bone loss during aging is also important. Milk has been of particular interest given calcium's integral role in bone health, with the majority of studies focusing on calcium itself and, later, vitamin D.

Thousands of studies have examined the role of calcium in bone health, hypothesizing that higher intakes build stronger bones, decrease bone losses and osteoporosis, and reduce fracture risk. While earlier research suggested a potential role for supplementation in decreasing osteoporosis and fractures, more recent studies including longer-term prospective studies and randomized controlled trials

(RCTs) do not support a clear association. One study also showed that the effect of calcium supplementation on fracture risk in women differed by site, with a 50% *increase* in hip fracture risk; this result was supported by additional observational data from the Study of Osteoporotic Fractures. And, even in healthy children actively accruing peak bone mass, the current evidence does not support a role for high intakes of calcium or supplementation for optimizing bone health.

Vitamin D is integral to calcium metabolism, as it maintains healthy blood calcium levels by increasing absorption of calcium from food or increasing resorption from bone. It has thus become a more recent focus of attention in terms of its role in bone health, either on its own or with calcium. A 2014 Cochrane review of 53 RCTs found that vitamin D alone was not effective at reducing fractures, a result found in other reviews, with fracture risk again varying by site. Many of these studies showed only a modest risk reduction even when taken with calcium. Some studies do indicate that supplements may be helpful among those with particularly low calcium and vitamin D intakes who may be deficient, however. Notably, calcium supplementation has also been associated with gastrointestinal distress, increased risk of renal disease, and even myocardial infarction, likely due to its broad set of biological activities beyond bone health. Yet no health risks are generally observed with calcium-rich foods, only with high-dose supplements.

Researchers have since turned their attention to milk and dairy foods in relation to bone health. A 2017 review notes that across the life cycle, from children to postmenopausal women, cow's milk, powdered milk supplements, and whey protein are all associated with a slower bone turnover, leading to either higher bone mineral density or no change. Yet few studies of milk on fracture risk have been performed, none of which are RCTs; and the results are equivocal, showing a higher, lower, or no relationship between milk and bone outcomes.

Are milk and dairy products related to obesity, prostate cancer, and other diseases?

Numerous studies have shown that consumption of milk and dairy products is not related to risk of weight gain or obesity in either children or adults as long as they're part of an energy-balanced diet. Some studies show that milk may even be helpful for weight loss, with whole milk showing stronger effects, perhaps in part because its extra fat provides greater satiety compared to nonfat milk. Other studies examining associations between milk and dairy and chronic diseases like T2DM and cardiovascular disease (CVD) show mixed findings, with most showing neutral and sometimes even favorable results. Associations with cancer have received much attention, as the estrogens and insulin-like growth factors (IGFs) in milk and dairy may play a role in initiating and promoting tumor development in hormone-sensitive cancers like those of the breast, endometrial system, ovaries, and prostate. (Although a number of studies demonstrate that biologically active estrogens in commercially available milk and dairy are too low to exert an adverse effect on human consumers.) Milk has been shown to stimulate the growth of prostate cancer cells in laboratory studies, for example, perhaps a result of its effects on plasma insulin and IGFs as well as cell signaling and growth, or of its whey and casein content. A few studies suggest that consumption of milk early in life, during growth and development, may be particularly harmful to healthy prostate development. For instance, a 2015 analysis of 32 prospective studies found that high intakes of total dairy products; milk, low- and nonfat milk; cheese; and total, dietary and dairy calcium, but not supplemental or nondairy calcium, were associated with an increased risk of prostate cancer. No associations were observed with individual foods like ice cream and butter, though whole milk was protective. These divergent results indicate that further studies are needed. There are certainly diet–gene interactions as well, with a recent review showing differing effects on prostate and other cancers in relation to different types of lactose intolerance.

In contrast to single food and food group studies of milk and dairy products, research on overall dietary patterns consistently shows that diets high in sweetened milk and dairy products like ice cream, yogurt, and flavored coffee drinks contribute added sugar to the diet, which increases the risk of T2DM and heart disease. Conversely, diet patterns that include reduced-fat milk and other low-fat dairy products are often related to less heart disease, lower obesity, and longer lifespan, likely because reduced-fat dairy products are often consumed as part of an overall healthy diet. At the same time, Mediterranean diets, which include low to moderate intakes of full-fat dairy products alongside a diet rich in plants and polyunsaturated fats from olives and nuts, show similar reductions in risk of diseases (though studies of prostate cancer itself are few). Indeed, emerging data suggest that whole-milk dairy products do not create a cardiovascular risk when consumed in moderation as part of an otherwise healthy diet, perhaps due to the nutrient-dense profile of dairy beyond its saturated fat content.

In sum, the research on the role of milk and dairy in health and disease prevention is quite complex, as it is for calcium and vitamin D in osteoporosis. Like many things in nutrition, individual foods, food groups, and nutrients considered in isolation may be less important to overall health and longevity: the whole diet is what matters most.

Why is yogurt unusual?

The discovery of yogurt may have been accidental, a product of milk transformation in the early years of animal domestication about 6000 years ago. Yogurt remains a part of many diets throughout the world still today, though how it's consumed differs across culture and cuisine. Turks and Indians sip yogurt-based drinks as a form of hydration and enjoyment, for example, the former seasoned with salt (ayran) and the latter with sugar and/or fruit (lassi). Those in the West are more likely to consume yogurt as breakfast, snack, or dessert, with Americans often opting for fruity versions heavily sweetened with added sugar.

Yogurt is made when live bacteria (e.g., *Lactobacillus bulgaricus, Streptococcus thermophilus, Lactobacillus acidophilus*) are added to milk, either with or without heat, producing lactic acid fermentation. The bacteria feed on milk's sugars and convert them to lactic acid, which gives yogurt its tang. Yogurt-making methods vary: "Greek" yogurt refers to its production process, not its location of origin, in which the mixture is strained to remove the (liquid) whey following fermentation; the method creates a thicker product that is higher in protein compared to thinner, American-style yogurts. Greek yogurt is common throughout eastern Europe, and strained yogurt in Iceland is called skyr. Drinkable kefir is common in Central Asia and some parts of Europe, in which added yeast (alongside bacteria) creates mild carbonation.

Yogurt contains many of the same nutrients found in milk, particularly protein, calcium, phosphorus, riboflavin, and vitamin B_{12}. Its claim to fame, however, is its bacteria. Though the salubrious effects of yogurt have been appreciated for millennia through observation and anecdote, it wasn't until 1908 that a Russian scientist first lauded its benefits, hypothesizing that longevity among Bulgarians was due to "good" bacteria in yogurt that crowded out pathogenic ("bad") bacteria throughout the digestive tract. Science has since shown that yogurt's effects are strain-specific and very much related to dose and frequency of consumption: physiological effects vary, and some strains do not survive digestive passage at all or fail to colonize in order to have a positive impact. Other strains provide "good" bacteria to the colon, an example of probiotics. Beneficial results are also notable in the stomach and small intestine: animal and laboratory models show that bacteria interact with intestinal epithelial cells, modifying the immune response to reduce inflammation and other conditions at the intestinal barrier that impact gut functioning and nutrient absorption. Lactic acid bacteria also reduce symptoms associated with lactose maldigestion due to their lactose-hydrolyzing enzymes. Some strains of bacteria are even able to synthesize several B vitamins. Good bacteria indeed!

There is strong evidence that yogurt improves and restores overall bowel function and reduces symptoms associated with conditions like gastroenteritis and inflammatory bowel syndrome (IBS). A 2014 review of 43 RCTs comparing probiotics with placebo, some of which were in the form of yogurt and other fermented milk products, reported a 21% reduction in IBS symptoms like abdominal pain and bloating; similar results were seen in a 2015 review. Some studies also suggest that yogurt can help control diarrhea resulting from antibiotic use, a common side effect of some medications. Health effects vary depending on the strain of bacteria, however.[2]

More recent studies have expanded research beyond the gut, though a clear health effect requires further investigation. A 2017 review found that only ten studies on obesity and weight gain had been conducted, for example, suggesting a beneficial effect, although results were inconsistent. Other studies have suggested protective effects for T2DM, with one study showing a 14% lower risk among yogurt consumers who ate 80–125 g/d. Yogurt eaters are likely to be healthier in other ways, however, including their overall diet, physical activity, and smoking behavior. Thus, RCTs are needed to better understand the independent health benefits of yogurt with specific control and calibration of bacterial strain. For instance, an analysis of 15 RCTs found that yogurt reduced low-density lipoprotein ("bad") cholesterol (LDL) significantly when consumption lasted 8 weeks or longer; *L. acidophilus* had the strongest effects, although those including multiple strains of bacteria were most effective.

Yogurt research today is exciting, with one recent RCT showing that yogurt with certain strains enhances natural killer cell activity, a key to immune function. And a few studies investigating the gut–brain axis have shown that yogurt can impact mental health and cognition, though many more studies are needed. It seems reasonable to surmise that yogurts made from plant-based milks like soy, almond, and coconut may provide the same benefits as dairy yogurts—again, it all depends on the strain(s) and dose of bacteria—though no such studies have yet been performed.

Are egg-white omelets the best choice for heart disease prevention?

The degree to which eggs played a role in Paleolithic diets is unknown, but production began in earnest during the Neolithic era, beginning with chicken domestication in Southeast Asia. Duck, goose, quail, and pigeon eggs later entered the diet. Much later, eggs gained popularity in the Middle Ages in Europe and are common today in many world cuisines.

Eggs are a relatively inexpensive source of protein; a large egg has 6 g with ~75 calories, 1.6 g of saturated fat, and 1.8 g of monounsaturated fat as well as iron, folate, and vitamins D, E, B_6, and B_{12}. Lutein and zeaxanthin, responsible for the sunshiny yolks, are carotenoids shown to reduce the risk of age-related macular degeneration in older adults, a condition that can lead to blindness. The yolks are also rich in choline, a mineral important in brain health and cognition.

Eggs are also particularly high in cholesterol, each one containing around 185 mg. Due to the recognized role of high blood cholesterol in heart disease, the 1968 American Heart Association recommended consuming less than 300 mg of dietary cholesterol daily and fewer than three whole eggs weekly. The guideline remained for years, leading to decreased egg consumption—and the rise of the egg-white omelet. Yet research has since shown that dietary cholesterol is not the main culprit responsible for elevating LDL, which is largely driven by trans fats and, to a far lesser degree, saturated fat (Chapter 8). Moreover, few studies had specifically examined the role of eggs in coronary heart disease (CHD). A seminal 1999 investigation in the Harvard prospective cohort studies found no significant association between egg consumption and risk of CHD or stroke, even at levels of five or six per week (the highest category). The study did show a two-fold increased risk of CHD among diabetic men and a 49% increase among women consuming one egg daily compared to one egg weekly, however. A number of other observational studies have since replicated these findings, and a 2013 analysis of 9 cohort studies also showed no significant association between egg consumption and CHD, with no trend for a higher risk for a one egg / day increase. That same analysis confirmed an amplified 54% increased risk of CHD among diabetics comparing highest to lowest egg consumers.

The surprising results in diabetics spurred several RCTs examining the impact of eggs on CHD risk factors (though none looked at CHD itself or myocardial infarction). A small study found no adverse effects on blood lipids comparing breakfasts with and without eggs in those with extant coronary artery disease. Another small study among overweight or obese people with T2DM or prediabetes found no significant differences in LDL or HDL and greater satiety among those consuming a high-egg diet (2 eggs/ day, 6 days/week) compared to fewer than 2 eggs /week. Thus, the possible risk of egg consumption on development of CHD among diabetics requires further investigation. Genetic studies will be helpful in clarifying whether eggs do increase CHD in some people. Even so, the 2015–2020 Dietary Guidelines for Americans no longer advises reducing egg consumption or limiting daily cholesterol intake to under 300 mg.

Are some eggs healthier and more sustainable than others?

There are more chickens in the world than any other bird: a stunning 50 billion chickens per year are raised for food globally. In the US alone, 50 billion eggs are produced annually. Meanwhile, eaters in the UK consume 33 million eggs daily.

Commercial egg production is dominated by CAFOs (aka, factory farming). Efficiency and cost are the dominant factors driving production, creating conditions as inhumane and troubling for laying hens as for other livestock. Hens are often housed in battery cages, which confine 4–12 birds with little room to move or spread their wings. Space per bird is around 67 square inches on average—less than a sheet of paper—although some "enhanced" cages increase the space to 116 inches. The cages are stacked in massive buildings, and the birds never leave their cages. Approximately 95% of eggs in the US come from caged chickens. During their average lifetime of 72 weeks, hens will produce about 320 eggs, a much quicker rate of production due to selective breeding and rearing conditions.

Alternatives exist, though choices are numerous and often unclear. A number of feel-good labels, like "all natural" (Chapter 4) and "farm fresh," have no meaning whatsoever—other than to get you to buy them. Yet others do say something about the production methods, as well as the nutritional content. Common practices include:

- **Cage-free:** Uncaged birds live in massive warehouses (aviaries) but do not go outdoors; they have around one square foot of space on average, though the amount varies; they are able to engage in some natural behaviors (e.g., walk, perch, spread their wings); crowding can cause unsanitary conditions and poor air quality, among other issues.
- **Free-range/free-roaming:** Uncaged birds have outdoor access, though the amounts of time and space vary greatly and may simply be a few doors leading to a cement pen outside, so many birds often don't go outside even if able.
- **Certified organic:** Eggs must come from free-range chickens and meet the standards of the USDA National Organic Program (Chapter 4), though practices vary.

- **Pasture-raised:** Uncaged birds spend most of their days outdoors and sleep in a barn at night; diets often include foods from their natural diets like worms and grass but may also be supplemented with corn; while space and conditions vary, many consider this to be the most humane production method.
- **Omega-3:** Feed is enriched with omega-3 fatty acids (Chapter 8) usually through the addition of flax meal or oil.
- **Pasteurized:** Pasteurizing eggs kills harmful pathogens, so they are safer and less likely to cause foodborne illness (Chapter 2).

Note that a number of these labels are not mutually exclusive, which is why cartons can get awfully crowded: some labels reflect production conditions; others, type of feed; still others, nutrification (Chapter 6). Regardless, the vast majority of commercial producers cut down the beaks of hens to prevent the birds from injuring themselves or other animals, which is otherwise common due to stress. They also induce "forced molting" through starvation to manipulate the laying cycle for production needs. These labels also tell little of what the hens ate, unless specified. "Vegetarian fed" is another common label, often used to convey that chickens are not fed animal byproducts, otherwise common in animal husbandry. Most commercially raised chickens are fed a corn-based diet—although chickens are omnivores that otherwise eat worms and insects.

Various certification programs are dedicated to animal welfare. The Animal Welfare Approved program has the highest standards and prohibits both beak cutting and forced molting. Other programs (e.g., Certified Humane, American Humane Certified, Food Alliance Certified) offer some protections but allow either beak cutting or molting. And the "United Egg Producers Certified" is simply the program for the egg industry, in which most hens are raised in either battery cages or "cage-free." (Hormones are not legally allowed in either poultry or egg production; antibiotics are commonly used in poultry, but not egg, production.)

If you're able, buying eggs from small, local farmers is one way to learn more easily about the source of your omelet: ask how the chickens are raised, what they're fed, if the eggs are pasteurized, whether the chickens live in cages and have outdoor access, and so forth. (Perhaps even ask if they're happy or have friends, if you like.) One delightful thing about local eggs, like other farmers market finds, is the wide variety. Brown eggs are common, yes, as are white. But so are blue. And green. (Green eggs are an actual thing, it turns out; and, unlike other colors, which only permeate the shell, the green pigment colors the entire egg and yolk. How fun is that?!) There are no differences in nutritional value between white and brown eggs, despite the myth that brown are healthier: they just come from different breeds, whose genetic variants lead to different colors, akin to hair or eye color in humans.[3]

While McDonald's may not serve green eggs and ham—of the more than 2 billion eggs they buy annually, the largest buyer in the US—the company announced in September 2015 that it would phase out purchasing eggs coming from battery cages and turn to cage-free eggs. The decision led 200 other companies to follow suit. While the use of cage-free eggs does eliminate confinement, it still allows CAFOs to continue.

13

WATER DWELLERS

FISH AND SEAFOOD

What are the nutritional benefits of seafood?

Like other animal foods, fish and shellfish are excellent sources of protein, as well as a number of B-complex vitamins, vitamin D, and minerals like iron, zinc, and selenium. There are five major categories of seafood. **Mollusks** (e.g., oyster, clam, mussel) are very low in calories, about ten per oyster; oysters provide omega-3 fatty acids, and mussels provide vitamin B_{12}. Mollusks are the lowest aquatic animals on the food chain and, thus, the most sustainable. Mollusks are also filter feeders that directly consume microscopic nutrients, organic matter, and phytoplankton, which in turn clean water. Oysters, for example, are a "keystone" species that restore ecosystems by decreasing excess nutrients, which can otherwise overload oceans due to pollution and contribute to dead zones (Chapter 2). **Crustaceans** (e.g., crab, shrimp, prawn, lobster, crayfish) are particularly rich in selenium, and pink-hued carotenoids like astazanthin give them their color; some have edible soft shells that provide calcium. **White fish** (e.g., sole, tilapia, hake, cod, halibut, pollock, flounder, catfish, swordfish) may be small and flat or large and round and are lean compared to fish like salmon, tuna, (lake) trout, arctic char, and bluefish. These **fatty fish** are the best sources of heart-healthy docasahexaenoic acid (DHA) and eicosapentaenoic acid (EPA) (Chapter 8), yet **small silver fish** (e.g., anchovy, herring, mackerel, sardine) have these essential fatty acids too—and their edible bones are also rich in calcium. (Sea vegetables and algae provide nourishment for many water-dwelling animals and are also wonderfully nutritious for humans [Chapter 9].)

Seafood has salutary effects throughout the body, particularly for cardiovascular disease (CVD); impacts on cognition and mental health and other health outcomes are promising but require more studies. While the World Health Organization (WHO) does not single out seafood as part of its dietary recommendations, it does highlight the importance of choosing protein-rich foods with unsaturated fats, like seafood, beans, legumes, and the like, over those with saturated fats, like red meat. Both British and American diet guidelines advise consuming at least two servings of seafood weekly and emphasize fatty fish due to its powerful marine fatty acids. Most individuals do not meet that goal, however, instead opting for beef, pork, and poultry. Further, Americans eat a limited range of seafood: nearly 75% of intake comes from shrimp, salmon, canned tuna, tilapia, and Alaskan pollock.

Does seafood prevent heart disease? What about "fish oil"?

Early investigations in the 1970s showed a lower risk of cardi-ovascular diseases in Eskimo and Inuit populations with high consumption of marine mammals. Associations were particularly strong for heart failure, and studies found a 15% lower risk when comparing highest to lowest consumers, with similar protection for marine omega-3 fatty acids DHA and EPA. Additional obser-vational studies confirmed these results, showing that eating fish once weekly had a similar reduction in fatal coronary heart dis-ease (CHD). At the same time, many observational studies began demonstrating a protective effect of seafood on other aspects of heart health, and research examining total dietary patterns that include seafood alongside other healthful foods showed similar results.

Early randomized controlled trials (RCTs) demonstrated that omega-3 supplementation reduced fatal cardiac events, leading the American Heart Association (AHA) to release a statement in 2002 recommending that those with CHD "consume ≈1 g/d EPA+DHA, preferably from oily fish, but EPA+DHA supplements could be considered in consultation with a physician." Note that the rec-ommendation is limited to people diagnosed with CHD because those were the individuals included in the RCTs. No RCTs had been conducted in groups of people free from CHD.

Studies since then have continued to examine the roles of sea-food, omega-3 fatty acids, and "fish oil" (omega-3 supplements) on CVD. Observational studies of both seafood and omega-3 intakes have continued to show beneficial effects on cardiovascular health, including in those free from heart disease. Yet subsequent RCTs examining the role of supplements have been inconsistent. Specifically, findings vary depending on the type of cardiovascular event and the people studied. And larger trials with longer follow-up, a general indicator of a higher-quality study, were less likely to show benefits. Yet well-designed RCTs examining those with extant heart disease generally indicated protective effects. Some scientists hypothesize that contradictory results are due in part to improved treatment and prevention of heart disease, whether through cholesterol-lowering statins or other measures managing heart health that may mask the role of (relatively subtle) dietary factors like omega-3 and fish oil. Doses may have also been too low to show a beneficial effect.

Based on the conflicting data since around 2003, the AHA reexamined the best available evidence to update the 2002 statement, if necessary. The report examined data from specific subgroups, including those at different levels of risk (e.g., those with and without T2DM). Ultimately, the AHA's 2002 advice remained largely unchanged: those with CHD should "consume ≈1 g/d EPA+DHA, preferably from oily fish, but EPA+DHA supplements could be considered." (Algae-based omega-3 supplements are now available for vegetarians, though they have not been examined in scientific studies.) Note the advice remains focused on "secondary prevention" to mitigate subsequent events, like a second heart attack, with data suggesting a possible 10% reduction in risk—and little possibility of harm. While there are some additional guidelines for those with specific clinical conditions, there are no current recommendations for intakes for "primary prevention" of heart disease in the general population (i.e., otherwise healthy, not at high risk of heart disease) as no trials in this group have yet been conducted. For those individuals, the best evidence still comes from observational studies, which continue to demonstrate the beneficial health effects of diets including seafood and omega-3s on preventing CVD.

What is the state of environmental contamination? Is seafood safe to eat?

There are numerous contaminants that get onto our plates from consuming seafood, so named "persistent, bioaccumulative, and toxic pollutants" (PBTs) in aggregate, also known as "persistent organic pollutants" (POPs). Common pollutants include mercury and methylmercury; dichlorodiphenyltrichloroethane (DDT), a pesticide banned in the US but still used elsewhere; polychlorinated biphenyls (PCBs) and dioxins, mainly from toxic waste; and polybrominated diphenyl ethers (PBDEs), found in flame retardants. While many of these occur to small degrees naturally, most are a result of industrial and manufacturing processes in which chemicals leach and/or are dumped directly into waterways and, over time, accumulate in seafood. Others are used in aquaculture (PCBs) or agriculture (DDT, Chapter 3, endnote 7).

Mercury is a neurotoxin POP with no smell or taste and leads to brain damage if consumed in large doses over a long duration. It occurs naturally in the environment but is also a heavy-metal byproduct of various industrial processes such as burning coal. It accumulates in oceans and waterways and is converted into methylmercury, its carbon-containing cousin found in the flesh of water-dwelling creatures. It's therefore found across almost all types of seafood, but the amount varies by species. Predatory fish—notably king mackerel, swordfish, shark (mako), tilefish (golden bass, golden snapper), and tuna—ingest smaller, contaminated species that have, in turn, consumed polluted phytoplankton. The mercury thus "bioaccumulates" in large fish species in far greater quantities compared to its prey, then reaches human eaters.

The mounting evidence of seafood contamination from mercury and other POPs over the past several decades, alongside heightened media attention and public awareness, has led to increased concern about consuming seafood. At the same time, nutrition science was showing the benefits of consuming seafood, particularly fish high in heart-healthy marine fatty acids.

Since then, studies concurrently examining the risks and benefits have illuminated whether seafood is safe to eat, what species, at what levels, and for whom. The current scientific consensus is that, for an average adult, the benefits of eating fish outweigh the risks when it comes to mercury. And regarding the risk of PCBs and dioxins, a striking study that reviewed and analyzed data from EPA and other organizations concluded that "if 100,000 people ate farmed salmon twice a week for 70 years, the extra PCB intake could potentially cause 24 extra deaths from cancer—but would prevent at least 7,000 deaths from heart disease." The Institute of Medicine used this and other studies to also conclude that the role of PCBs in cancer is negligible from a public health perspective. And both the Food and Agriculture Organization of the United Nations (FAO) and WHO drew similar conclusions: the risk of potential cancer from PCB and dioxin exposure is far outweighed by the benefit of decreased risk of CHD.

A sign of good news: a 2016 study by scientists at Scripps Institution of Oceanography showed that global contamination of wild seafood has been decreasing in recent years. The group examined studies from 1969 to 2012 to evaluate the scope, magnitude, and variability across a range of PBTs and showed declines ranging from 15% to 30% per decade across all categories, a result of effective water pollution–mitigation programs.

Is seafood healthy for pregnant and breastfeeding women and young children?

Pregnant and breastfeeding women have specific nutritional needs. Marine omega-3s DHA and EPA are critical in cell membranes throughout the body, especially in the brain and eyes. But mercury has an exceptionally toxic effect in babies, and high exposure in utero and in newborns can cause irreparable brain damage. Yet even among this vulnerable group research has shown that seafood is a healthy part of a diet for new moms and young children. In fact, young children who didn't consume adequate EPA and DHA performed worse on tests of visual acuity and cognition later in life in some studies. Even so, mothers have stringent dietary guidelines regarding seafood consumption because of mercury's grave effects. Consensus from several professional health organizations pertaining to pregnant and nursing women and young children, including the most recent 2017 guidelines issued jointly by FDA and USDA is:

- **Do eat** *either* (1) 2–3 servings weekly of a variety of "best choices" lower in mercury, including fatty fish (e.g., salmon, catfish, sardine, flounder, tilapia, oyster) and canned light tuna— skipjack is the smallest, most plentiful, least contaminated species often used in canned tuna—**or** (2) 1 serving weekly of "good choices," which have somewhat higher mercury content (e.g., bluefish, grouper, mahi mahi, albacore and yellowfin tuna, snapper). Sushi, which is often yellowfin tuna, is controversial, mainly because it is raw and thus carries a greater risk of foodborne illness—though some scientists believe it can be enjoyed on occasion.
- **Do eat** a variety of fish.
- **Avoid/do not eat** any fish with the highest levels of mercury, including swordfish, king mackerel, shark, orange roughy (from the Gulf of Mexico), tilefish (aka, golden bass, golden snapper), or bigeye tuna.
- **Be careful** concerning fish caught by friends and family from local waterways like rivers and lakes (e.g., carp, catfish, trout, perch). Do not eat more than once per week, if at all, since pollution is often greater, contamination is more severe, and safe levels for consumption may be unknown. Consult state advisories for specific advice on locally caught fish before consuming, and if none is provided, eat only once weekly and no other seafood that week.

The 2017 guidelines can be found online in a one-page, user-friendly list designed for everyday eaters that includes many specific examples. The overarching message is that "fish and other protein-rich foods have nutrients that can help your child's growth and development." The guidelines may be overly conservative for children, however, due to their focus on mercury: the 2017 guidelines recommend children 2 years and older should consume 1–2 servings of seafood weekly following the same guidelines as above. Yet there is some research to show that seafood can be consumed along with other solid foods beginning around 6 months of age, not only for the previously noted benefits in terms of vision and IQ but also to reduce the risk of developing seafood allergies.

Research on exposure and neurotoxicity of mercury continues given its potent effect on infant development. A 2014 report examined 164 studies of women and infants from 43 countries around the world to compare hair and blood mercury levels by seafood consumption in comparison to FAO reference levels. High seafood consumers in Arctic regions and those living near gold-mining regions had levels well over the threshold, while those in coastal regions of Southeast Asia and the western Pacific and Mediterranean were below (but approaching) the reference. We must continue to monitor mercury levels in oceans, waterways, and seafood consumers around the world to ensure that levels do not cause cognitive impairment—particularly in light of the increasing focus on seafood as a contributor to healthy diets.

What are the benefits and risks of aquaculture?

Global fish consumption per capita has increased around 3.2% annually, from 9.9 kg in the 1960s to 19.7 kg in 2013. Throughout human history the vast majority of seafood has come from catch fisheries, defined by FAO as "A unit determined by an authority or other entity that is engaged in raising and/or harvesting fish . . . defined in terms of some or all of the following: people involved, species or type of fish, area of water or seabed, method of fishing, class of boats, and purpose of the activities." Yet the confluence of increased seafood demand and decreased wild supplies due to exploitation, pollution, and depletion of catch fisheries (Chapter 2) has revolutionized the way seafood is procured. While the numbers of animals from catch fisheries have remained relatively constant since the late 1980s, aquaculture (analogous to terrestrial agriculture) has shown tremendous growth: about 50% of seafood now comes from aquaculture production, climbing over the years from 7% in 1974 to 26% in 1994 and 39% in 2004. Though the vast majority of aquaculture efforts are related to animals, there is a far smaller but growing market for sea vegetables and plants.

Aquaculture has been around for millennia, beginning in Egypt around 2500 BCE and later emerging in China and North Africa. France began cultivating mollusks in 600 BCE, while Japan began producing seaweed in 400 CE. Aquaculture methods and processes developed over the centuries following improvements in tools and mechanization, just like agriculture. Intensive rainbow trout farming took off in Europe in the 1960s, followed by Atlantic salmon. Today, FAO defines aquaculture as "the farming of aquatic organisms, including fish, mollusks, crustaceans, and aquatic plants" that "implies some form of intervention in the rearing process to enhance production, such as regular stocking, feeding, protection from predators, etc." as well as "individual or corporate ownership of the stock being cultivated." The latter clause is significant, FAO asserts, as it denotes the difference from wild aquatic organisms that do not technically belong to any one person or entity.

The National Oceanic and Atmospheric Association divides aquaculture into two types. **Marine aquaculture** produces ocean species, primarily oysters, clams, mussels, shrimp, and salmon but also cod, sea bass, sea bream, yellowtail tuna, and barramundi either in the ocean (often in cages, on the seafloor, or in a water column) or in ponds or tanks. **Freshwater aquaculture** takes place primarily in ponds or tanks and produces river, lake, and stream species, primarily catfish in the US but also bass, tilapia, and trout. As in agriculture, there are diverse feeding and confinement and waste management systems used in aquaculture. FAO further describes aquaculture as **extensive**, which works in concert with natural stocks and production; **intensive** (and **hyperintensive**), which requires high-level inputs for fertilization, disease control, feeding, manipulating stocks, and harvesting to maximize growth and efficiency; and **semi-intensive**, which falls somewhere in between. Aquaculture can also be divided into subsistence, artisanal, specialized, or industrial according to the level of intensification, resources, and the consumer market.

Because intensification is a continuum, the specific farming practices employed are paramount when considering sustainability. There are fed and nonfed species in aquaculture, the latter of which do not require feed because they are filter feeders (e.g., oysters)—and what farmed fish eat impacts the environmental footprint. As well, systems may be based on water (e.g., cages, pens, inshore/offshore) or land (natural or irrigated ponds, tanks, raceways), recycling (highly controlled and enclosed or open recirculation with surrounding waters) or integrated (including both livestock and fish). The story of farmed salmon is exemplary: as wild Atlantic salmon populations were being decimated due to high consumer demand, novel aquaculture methods allowed farmed salmon to thrive in northern Europe and Scandinavia, particularly Norway, which decreased the threats from humans to wild salmon. In time, wild salmon populations began to recover, preserving the species to swim another day.

Today, farmed salmon accounts for about 70% of global supply—the fastest-growing food production system in the world, according to the World Wildlife Fund (WWF)—and the major consumers are Americans. But early farming practices, and still some today, were questionable regarding social and environmental impacts: salmon were fed using fish oil or meal made from small silver fishes, which imbalances those species in wild populations and disrupts aquatic ecosystems; some feed was contaminated with toxins, which entered the food supply; wastewater was discharged into open waters, including excrement and antibiotic residues; and some fish escaped. (Fish on the run reached a new level of concern in 2017, when genetically engineered [GE] salmon escaped from their pen, though they were later caught.) Improper temperature and other rearing conditions to increase growth rate also led to skeletal deformities and spinal disorders in some salmon farms. Further, the use of chemicals in aquaculture, including pesticides, antibiotics, and the like, has the same potential for ill effects on the animals raised, the environment, and farmworkers.

Indeed, many of the problems faced by aquaculture are not much different from those in agriculture, with many like-minded groups emerging to demand environmentally conscious production. It's worth noting that salmon farming and other finfish aquaculture is still generally more sustainable than raising terrestrial animals: farmed fish produces lower overall greenhouse gas emission (GHGe), uses less land and water, and has a higher feed conversion efficiency. Yet the overall environmental footprint will grow substantially over time in light of the skyrocketing aquaculture industry, and converting feed into fish is far more resource-intensive and less efficient than consuming the plants (or smaller animals) that fed them.

The rising awareness of the environmental concerns regarding farmed salmon incited a backlash, and the industry has been cleaning itself up and becoming more sustainable. The Aquaculture Stewardship Council (ASC) was jointly formed in 2004 by The Netherlands and UK and envisions a world "where aquaculture plays a major role in supplying food and social benefits for mankind whilst minimizing negative impacts on the environment." In 2010, the nonprofit thus set seven standards for salmon farming and eleven other species: (1) Protect ecosystems and preserve biodiversity; (2) Control antibiotic use and reduce the use of pesticides and other chemicals; (3) Prevent escapes that can contaminate wild fish through spread of parasites; (4) Regulate feed practices and confirm sustainability; (5) Preserve water quality; (6) Protect endangered sites; and (7) Guard worker rights and safety through fair wages and conditions and prohibit child slavery. Fifteen salmon farming companies, representing 70% of global production, later formed the Global Salmon Initiative, with the intent to fully meet the ASC Salmon Standard by 2020.

Despite these gains, new problems continually arise, as in any farming operation. Sea lice infested more than half of Scotland's farmed salmon populations in 2017, for example, a problem virtually unheard of 30 years ago. Sea lice have become a growing problem around the world. Pesticides and antibiotics are employed to address the threat, though the lice are becoming more resistant, forcing the use of increasingly toxic chemicals and inhumane methods to combat the condition. Production has decreased, costs have risen, and residues from wastewater have ended up in waterways.

Even so, many scientists, governmental organizations, nonprofits, and international nongovernmental organizations like FAO, WHO, and others believe that aquaculture is critical to reducing poverty and improving food security and nutrition around the world. Subsistence and rural aquaculture for household consumption and/ or income in impoverished communities is deemed essential to this end. Time will tell if farming aquatic animals proves less damaging to the environment than terrestrial farming while still successfully meeting the food and nutrition needs of those in the developing world—or whether aquaculture is truly necessary to feed the population in 2050, as many maintain. It all depends on the species, particularly its place in the food chain, as well as the specific practices employed. And, despite the gains in technology, production, and sustainability during the past several decades, much work remains to be done—and individuals most in need of protein-rich seafood, like those in sub-Saharan Africa and Asia, are yet to benefit significantly from aquaculture.

14

WATER, COFFEE, AND TEA

IMPACTS ON HEALTH AND ENVIRONMENT

Why is water essential for life, and how much do we need?

Water is the sixth essential nutrient required for life. Our bodies are approximately 60% water, about 75% in infants and 55% in older adults, which is critical for numerous bodily processes. Blood is mainly water, and it transports oxygen and vitamins and minerals to cells and organs and removes waste products. Cells are also mainly water—two-thirds of total body water is intracellular—facilitating chemical reactions, cell-to-cell communication, and cell division and apoptosis (cell death). The other fluids in our bodies are also mainly water (e.g., cerebrospinal, synovial, ocular), providing lubrication for each organ and system. Fluid homeostasis is integrally related to and regulated by electrolytes like sodium and potassium (Chapter 7) that impact how efficiently our hearts beat and pump blood; imbalances are fatal if unaddressed. Humans can survive for weeks without food, but the human body will shut down completely after around 72 hours without water, though survival may last a week or more under comfortable, temperate conditions for a healthy adult. Whereas our body carries with it a store of energy for power, slowly broken down as needed during food shortages, water must be replaced consistently as it is lost daily through normal metabolic processes such as respiration, perspiration, and elimination.

So essential is hydration to health that our brains generally let us know when we need water. Through intricate organ-to-organ, cell-to-cell communication, the need for water will eventually reach our brain, signaling a feeling of thirst. In other words, we don't

need an app for that. (Yes, it exists.) And there is no need to drink
eight glasses of water daily as such. The advice sounds sensible, but
there is no research behind this adage. The most recent Institute of
Medicine report estimated daily water needs at about 91 ounces (11+
cups) for women and 125 ounces (15+ cups a day) for men. Happily,
approximately 20% of this need is met by water-rich food like fruits,
vegetables, and dairy: watermelon is 92% water, lettuce is 95%, and
yogurt is 85%, for example. Beverages meet the remaining 80%.
Thus, about 3 liters of water (13 cups) for men and 2.2 liters (9 cups)
for women remain. Coffee, tea, fruit juice, soda, and beer can all contribute to hydration as all contain water. Earlier research suggested
that caffeine and alcohol have diuretic effects, but studies now show
that despite an initial increase in urination following consumption,
the effects are minimal and short-lasting. (Though alcohol's effects
vary depending on the type and how it is served: ethanol does de-
press an antidiuretic hormone that can lead to higher fluid losses
through urine than what is gained through consumption in some
cases.) Individual water needs depend on factors like sex, age, climate (e.g., heat and humidity), body composition, and physical activity. Metabolic factors affecting perspiration are important as sweat
is a big component of water loss. These differences impact how much
you need to drink, though the human body is generally excellent at
signaling when total body water is imbalanced via thirst.

Even so, some may need assistance maintaining healthy hydration. Older adults may neglect to drink water, whether due to habit,
desensitized thirst signal recognition, or cognitive impairments;
they also urinate more frequently. Children are also at greater risk
for dehydration due to such factors as inability to articulate water
needs (when very young). Illnesses and diseases associated with
high temperatures or water losses (like diarrhea or vomiting) are
also risk factors for dehydration. Hydration during serious and
prolonged physical activity (e.g., elite athlete, military) is complicated because increased sweating also increases loss of electrolytes,
which are critical for cell and blood volume. Professional and serious athletes thus often create a hydration schedule to ensure that
fluid and electrolyte needs are met but not exceeded. Dehydration
can be fatal—but so can water intoxication (and associated
hyponatremia, or low blood sodium concentration), although this
is extremely rare.

What are the differences between tap and bottled water?

Research since the mid-20th century has shown that fluoridated water decreases tooth decay by at least 25% in communities where employed. Indeed, the Centers for Disease Control and Prevention lists fluoridation as 1 of the 10 great public health achievements of the 20th century (!). Fluoridated water at concentrations between 0.5 and 1.5 mg/liter, adapted to the baseline fluoride intake of the population being served, helps build stronger teeth and prevents dental caries in children in particular. Opponents of fluoridation have cited risks ranging from birth defects to cancers, though there is no scientific evidence to support these claims. Still, like all nutrients, the poison is in the dose, and extremely high fluoride intakes (6–14 mg/liter daily) can lead to tooth and skeletal fluorosis (weaker teeth and bones); such conditions are rare, extremely unlikely, and far beyond the doses used in public health fluoridation projects. (Although those with clinically diagnosed renal malfunction with impaired fluoride metabolism should consult a physician.)

Bottled water can be a lifesaver in many situations, particularly in places where drinking water is unsafe or inaccessible; the former situation can be handled efficiently and cost-effectively in many cases through filters (or water purification tablets, in some settings). Yet drinking bottled water became trendy in the late 20th century, and intake has quadrupled since the 1990s. In 2015, about half of all Americans occasionally or mainly turned to bottled water in lieu of the tap. And we've been inundated with bottled waters of all kinds, including those nutrified (e.g., with electrolytes) at a premium price, or claiming superior taste and pristine sources which are often little more than marketing gimmicks. In some accounts, the source of bottled water has been mislabeled to mislead consumers.

An astonishing 50 billion bottles of water were consumed in 2015 in the US alone, and use is skyrocketing in Asia. A 2016 report from the Ellen MacArthur Foundation, the World Economic Forum, and McKinsey & Company estimated that by 2050 the Earth's oceans will contain more plastic by weight than fish (!) and bottles are a major contributor.

But copious research has shown that bottled water is no more nutritious than tap, on average, and vitamin- and mineral-enhanced waters are unnecessary for most people. Those drinking bottled water in all likelihood obtain more than enough micronutrients through the diet already, and the excess is simply excreted. (Thus, you are just creating expensive urine, pissing away your money.) Bottled water may also include contaminants, if improperly processed; and some chemicals used in packaging have been shown to leach into the water in some studies. And blind taste tests comparing both expensive and inexpensive bottled waters with tap have indicated that tap was just as tasty—and, in some studies, preferred.

Beyond all of this is the tremendous costs and waste arising from bottled water. The (ironic) cost of creating bottled water is substantial and ranges from 3 to 7 liters of water to create a 1-liter plastic bottle, depending on the variables included in the calculation; the most conservative estimate is 1.39 liters for a 1-liter water bottle, or 39% more than what's inside. And it takes about 2000 times more energy to produce, transport, and refrigerate bottled water compared to twisting the tap. Plastic bottles are usually made from polyethylene terephthalate (aka, Pet), which is estimated to take around 400 years to decompose, though the material is highly recyclable— but only 32% of Americans do so. Globally, that proportion is about 14% (which also includes similar plastics), and another 14% is burned. Recycling still requires energy, although fewer greenhouse gases (GHGs) are emitted compared to those coming from landfills, which is where about 40% of plastic bottles end up.[1] Interestingly, China's landfills are bereft of plastic bottles since they are regathered for recycling as a national cost- (if not environment-) saving effort.

The remaining 32% of plastics, many of which come from bottled water, are "mismanaged," and the vast majority end up in the ocean. Approximately 8 million metric tons of plastic are added annually, contributing to the 110 metric tons already there. Much of the plastic ends up being broken into tiny pieces over time, which are then consumed by ocean dwellers and seabirds mistaking it for food. Some studies have shown that high seafood consumers have detectable levels of plastics in their body. The larger pieces aggregate in gargantuan garbage piles known as "gyres"; the two largest are in the North Pacific and Atlantic oceans. Astonishingly, environmental scientists estimate that only about 1% of the waste is located in these gyres; thus, the rest has sunk, been consumed, or frozen. Another hypothesis is that microbes digest the plastic waste, which yield toxic byproducts like polychlorinated biphenyls (PCBs).

Can drinking water help with weight loss, or prevent kidney stones?

It has been hypothesized that sipping water throughout the day, and especially drinking a glass or two before a meal, can facilitate weight loss. Evidence is lacking, however, in part because water is so quickly absorbed following ingestion. Yet when water supplants caloric beverages like soda, fruit juice, and milk, the resultant lower energy intake by 10–13% can produce weight loss. Water also affects physiological parameters like energy expenditure and fat oxidation that can theoretically impact weight. Effects vary, depending on factors like baseline weight and diet composition; thus, more research is needed to determine the specific conditions in which water can be effective for weight loss and weight maintenance. However, water-rich foods that increase stomach volume on fewer calories— like soups, stews, and the like—are strongly associated with lower energy intake and weight loss in a wide range of individuals.

Water is particularly important for kidney function. Higher urine output due to increased fluid intake has been related to the prevention and lower recurrence of kidney stones in several meta-analyses and systematic reviews that included randomized controlled trials (RCTs). Protective effects were observed for water, coffee, alcohol, and tea but not sugary, caffeinated, or dairy beverages; effects with coffee, tea, and alcohol may be related to phytochemical and physiological effects found in these beverages beyond their hydrating effects.

How are coffee and caffeine unique?

Europeans have been enjoying coffee far longer than Americans and consume it in much higher quantities. Finns had the highest coffee consumption in the world per capita in 2014, quaffing down 1252 cups per year on average compared to a mere 369 cups in the US. *Coffea arabica* and *Coffea canephora* (var. *robusta*) are the two major coffee crops in commercial production, though the preferred flavor of arabica dominates world trade (80%). Brazil is the world's leading coffee producer.

Coffee contains more than 1000 known phytochemicals that contribute to its (sublime) sensory properties, as well as its health effects. It is a top source of antioxidant polyphenols in the diet, providing more than any other plant food; and its chlorogenic acids caffeic and ferulic acid feed "good" gut bacteria (Chapter 4). Yet there is considerable variability in the biological activity of coffee due to differences in species and geographic origin; production, postharvest, and storage practices; roasting process and degree; slow-brew or instant; and brewing method (boil, filter, espresso). Many of these factors also impact caffeine content, one of coffee's major claims to fame, which ranges from 95 to 330 mg in 8 fluid ounces of brewed drip coffee (and 30–70 mg in instant).

It is because of coffee's varied chemicals and effects on health that support has ranged from yay to nay over the years. Early studies focused only on caffeine, which is just one of coffee's many components, and extrapolated (erroneously, despite the high correlation) from those findings to coffee as a beverage. Caffeine is the most commonly consumed psychoactive drug in the world, a stimulant found in more than 60 plants. And coffee is the most frequent supplier of caffeine to the diet. Caffeine has been shown to enhance physical performance and endurance in athletes and the military and to improve concentration, memory, cognition, alertness, and focus; similar effects have been shown in the general population, perhaps why so many head straight to the coffee pot each morning. Coffee and caffeine can negatively impact sleep quantity and quality, especially in older adults, who generally have greater sensitivity to caffeine. Effects on sleep in younger people vary, in part due to genetic polymorphisms related to caffeine metabolism. Scientists Clark and Landolt point out in their 2017 review, however, that research on coffee, caffeine, and sleep is far more limited than one might expect—and has mostly been conducted among white European men. Thus, more studies in diverse populations are needed.

Because of caffeine's varied mechanisms in the body, studies have shown both positive and negative impacts. For example, impacts on blood pressure are in part a function of whether effects were measured directly after drinking or whether or not one was a habitual consumer (reflecting potential drug tolerance). An analysis of RCTs found that while caffeine on its own increased blood pressure, coffee had the opposite effect, likely due to its many other chemicals (like polyphenols and minerals) that have anti-inflammatory and other effects that decrease blood pressure. In a different set of studies beginning in the 1980s, coffee was shown to increase low-density lipoprotein ("bad") cholesterol (LDL), a risk factor for heart disease. Later research suggested, however, that this effect, attributed to coffee's phytochemical diterpenes cafestol and kahweol, varies greatly by coffee preparation: boiled coffee such as Turkish, Greek, and French press retains these LDL-increasing components, while filtered brewing removes them. We now know that genetics plays a role in the cardiometabolic effects of caffeine too: a 2015 study among European and African American adults identified eight genetic loci associated with habitual coffee consumption that were located near genes related to caffeine metabolism, for example.

How is coffee related to heart health and type 2 diabetes?

It is easy to lose the forest for the trees when it comes to coffee's health effects: there are simply too many unique components, which vary based on factors that aren't always considered. Nutritional and clinical studies that study the whole brew are helpful since that's the way coffee is usually consumed. Epidemiologic studies in particular are also able to account for some of the differences in coffee preparation that can otherwise obfuscate results. Findings from these studies are particularly strong for cardiovascular benefits. A 2014 meta-analysis of 36 prospective cohort studies with more than 1.2 million participants found that those drinking 3–5 cups of coffee daily had the lowest risk of cardiovascular disease (CVD) compared to nondrinkers. While protective effects were not observed at higher intakes, those drinking 6 or more cups did not have an increased risk. An investigation by the same team found that those consuming 1 cup a day were 8% less likely than nondrinkers to develop T2DM, which increased to 21% for 3 cups and 33% for 6 cups. Similar, though somewhat weaker, findings were observed for decaf coffee drinkers. The differences in findings between effects on heart disease and T2DM may be explained in part by caffeine's detrimental effect on heart health in high amounts in some people, whereas protection from diabetes is likely due to phytochemical activity (like chlorogenic acids) and minerals related to improved blood sugar and insulin sensitivity, not just caffeine.

Caffeine Caution

Caffeine is a drug, and consumption of this stimulant can lead to deleterious effects on blood pressure, heart rate, and sleep. Excessive intake may cause headaches, nausea, anxiety, and restlessness in some; the quantities leading to these effects vary among humans due to genetic and other factors (e.g., age, sex, weight, tolerance). Pregnant women should not consume caffeine (hence caffeinated coffee) in appreciable amounts, if at all, due to potential negative impacts on fetal growth and increased risk of spontaneous abortion. Caffeine is also physically addictive and dangerous at excessive amounts for some people, and withdrawal effects (like headaches, irritability, and fatigue) may occur. Decaf coffee has lower amounts of polyphenols and minuscule amounts of caffeine, around 3–12 mg per 8 fluid ounces, but has been shown to have some of the same health benefits as regular coffee in some studies. The evidence base is weaker because relatively few people consume decaffeinated coffee, which limits statistical power to detect an association in many studies.

Coffee Caveat

The overall health benefits that coffee brings dwindle once cream and sugar—and that includes flavored syrups and so forth—are added. (But you already knew that, right?)

Is coffee beneficial for other diseases, like depression?

There has been a resurgence in coffee research, with scientists hypothesizing protective effects on such conditions as liver disease, gallbladder disease, cancer, obesity, and depression. Research is strong that coffee is protective for a wide range of liver diseases and improves liver functioning even among those with extant disease. There is also growing evidence that both coffee and caffeine are protective for depression. A 2016 meta-analysis of 11 observational studies showed that coffee was linearly related to a decreased risk of depression, with a 17% lower risk among those consuming 4–5 cups daily compared with nondrinkers. A nonlinear association was observed with caffeine itself, with protective effects increasing from

68 to 509 mg/day but decreasing thereafter. These effects are consistent with the pharmacology of caffeine, which is a drug known to boost mood. However, benefits dwindle at high doses due to negative side effects. The impact of coffee and caffeine on neurodegenerative conditions like Parkinson's and Alzheimer's as well as dementia appears promising, though too few studies have been conducted to show a conclusive relationship. Two very large studies in 2017, one including more than 450 000 people across 10 countries in Europe and one set in the US, found that coffee was also related to greater longevity: men consuming the highest amount of coffee had a 12% lower risk of death (that is, death from all causes), and women had a 7% lower risk; significantly reduced risks were also observed for diseases of the digestive, cardiovascular, circulatory, and cerebrovascular systems.

Taken together, much of the recent clarity on coffee's health effects is due to a shift in how scientists conceptualize and measure diet. In this case, conflating "caffeine" with "coffee" can be misleading: coffee contains thousands of different components that have independent effects unrelated to caffeine. Reducing "coffee" to "caffeine" is another example of reductionism that has plagued nutrition and medical research. Caffeine is a powerful drug, but the whole (cup of coffee) is greater than the sum of its parts. Furthermore, coffee is consumed as part of an overall dietary pattern—and it is this everyday way of eating that is more important than any single component when it comes to a lifetime of good health and disease prevention.

What's behind coffee production?

Coffee is the second highest traded commodity in the world, right after crude oil. This crop, like others, traditionally employs production methods that damage the environment. Forests are cleared to plant coffee beans, often as a single crop. This negatively impacts biodiversity, compromises soil health, and removes a carbon sink that helps reduce the buildup of carbon in the atmosphere. (In contrast, "shade-grown" coffee is planted underneath trees, which is beneficial for ecosystems and preserves soil health.) Copious pesticides are often used in coffee production, further damaging the land. As well, coffee farmers are often undercompensated and exploited, earning little for such a cherished crop.

All of these factors have contributed to a consumer movement that demands more sustainably and ethically grown coffee that protects the environment and treats farmers fairly, evidenced by the myriad labels gracing many of today's coffee packages.

Organic coffee refers simply to the production methods (Chapter 4), but that is just the beginning. "Rainforest Alliance Certified" coffee is committed to environmental sustainability; "Fair Trade International" supports cooperatives of small farmers with a fair wage; and "Bird Friendly" (Smithsonian Migratory Bird Center), the most rigorous program, protects biodiversity through organic, shade-grown coffee. Many businesses have their own programs, like Starbucks: "C.A.F.E. (Coffee and Farmer Equity) Practices" encourages both environmental and ethical practices—though most aren't organic.

Few coffee producers and distributors do all things for all causes. Nevertheless, there are more ways than ever before for today's eco- and socially conscious coffee lovers to put their morning routine to good.

What are the main types of tea? What is kombucha?

Tea is the most popular beverage in the world next to water. Tea leaves have antimicrobial properties, and tea is also a safer beverage compared to unclean drinking water as boiling kills many pathogens. Tea originated in China c.2737 BCE and was consumed for its purported medicinal effects as well as for hydration, enjoyment, and ritual. It became a favored drink in England in the 17th century and was then disseminated throughout the British colonies, particularly India. China still produces most of the world's tea. India is second and is the creator of the beloved chai, a spicy-sweet tea blend with milk.

True teas are made from dried leaves grown in temperate regions around the world. In places like India, people (mostly women) can be seen stooped over on the hillside picking tea, back-breaking and difficult work under the hot sun. Eight different teas are created from *Camellia sinensis*, which vary in color, flavor, caffeine content, and phytonutrient content. Teas are left to dry, which leads to oxidation (i.e., the leaves age, water evaporates, and more oxygen is absorbed). Some teas can become naturally fermented due to microbial action if left out for long periods of time. Tea species, climate, cultivation, and processing method also affect these factors.

There are five main types of tea: (1) **Black:** fully ripened tea leaves are oxidized, dried, and withered and become black, though less oxidized teas have browner hues; (2) **Oolong** (aka, wulong): dried, withered, and twisted tea leaves are partially oxidized, hence reddish-brown; (3) **Green:** immature tea leaves are dried and steamed, yielding little oxidation and a light green color; (4) **White:** youngest tea shoots (buds) with white leaf hairs are unoxidized and white in color; and (5) **Pu-erh:** older tea plants with tender tea leaves are semioxidized and aged, leading to natural fermentation that produces beneficial bacteria; it is often darkest in color. Of these, black is the most commonly consumed tea globally (78%), followed by green (20%) and oolong (2%); black is preferred in the West and green in the East. Pu-erh is consumed mainly in China.

True tea only comes from tea leaves, yet many use the word to describe any beverage made from hot water and dried plants. Herbal "teas" are common, like those made from dried peppermint. It's also easy to find fruited teas (with or without herbs) and teas made from dried flowers, like rosebud, chamomile, or hibiscus. Pure herbal "tea" does not include tea leaves and thus provides different nutritional benefits consistent with its components. As well, the plants used to make herbal tea don't have caffeine, so herbal tea is naturally decaffeinated. Many regions refer to beverages that don't contain tea leaves as "infusions" or "tisanes" to avoid obfuscation. Peppermint tea, for example, can refer to either a decaffeinated herbal infusion or black tea flavored with peppermint essence, the latter of which *is* caffeinated. Read labels carefully to prevent a sleepless night, and ask servers in restaurants to provide the tea bag as many are unaware of the differences. (**Yerba maté** [maté], popular in South America, is made from the holly plant—neither tea nor herbs—and does have caffeine as well as a rich array of vitamins and phytochemicals.)

Kombucha is the newest tea craze to hit the US, though it and other fermented beverages have been part of traditional diets in such places as China, Russia, and Germany for millennia. Kombucha is made by brewing black tea and adding so-called SCOBY (symbiotic culture of bacteria and yeast) along with sugar, which creates fermentation. The chemical reactions produce carbonation and nutritional components like B-complex vitamins, as well as a host of organic acids that impart its sour taste. Fermentation also leads to the production of alcohol, and various processing methods manage the reaction and ingredients to enhance or reduce the final alcoholic content (think cider as a nonalcoholic fruit juice served to kids versus an adult beverage that ranges in alcohol content). Elements like herbs may be added for flavor, such as sugar for sweetness or probiotics (i.e., "good" bacteria, Chapter 4) to enhance healthfulness. For all of these reasons and others, kombucha products vary greatly: reading the nutrition facts panel and ingredients is essential.

While kombucha has reached "superfood" status with some health enthusiasts, there is little research to support the myriad commercial (and anecdotal) claims of its effects, though studies are underway. Conversely, kombucha can be a health hazard, whether due to unsafe preparation like a lack of pasteurization (Chapter 4) or as a source of added sugar and extra calories. A few studies have also shown that kombucha consumed in excess may even carry serious risks like metabolic acidosis or liver damage, though such effects are rare.

What are tea's nutritional and health benefits— and how is green tea distinctive?

Tea contains six classes of flavonoids, mainly catechins, as well as anthocyanins and other phytochemicals. Many have antioxidant, anticarcinogenic, antimutagenic, antimicrobial, and anti-inflammatory activity. Caffeine and theanine (an amino acid) are also found in tea, along with vitamin C. Green tea has a higher concentration of catechins (about 30–40% by weight) compared to black tea (~10%) and is also higher in vitamin C and theanine. Cell culture and animal studies indicate that green tea extracts have wide-ranging effects on metabolic, cognitive, neurological, and cardiovascular outcomes, stimulating a growing body of research in humans.

The strongest evidence of green tea's beneficial effects on health have been shown for blood pressure, especially among those with hypertension, as well as LDL cholesterol. The greatest impacts were seen among those with a mean systolic blood pressure of 130 mm Hg or more and among those consuming green tea as an extract. Of note, many studies have also shown similar effects for black tea. While more RCTs with larger sample sizes are needed, a meta-analysis of 22 prospective studies also found that an increase in any tea consumption by 3 cups per day was related to significantly lower risks of coronary heart disease (27%), stroke (18%), and mortality (24%). More recently, a smaller meta-analysis of 9 studies supported these findings, showing that those drinking 1–3 cups of green tea daily had a reduced risk of myocardial infarction (19%) and stroke (36%) compared to those who drank less than 1 cup per day. The effect was even stronger among those drinking at least 4 cups per day, demonstrating a 32% decreased risk of myocardial infarction.

Findings on the role of green tea in cancer are mixed, as they are for so many dietary components due to the diverse biology of cancer development in different parts of the body. While some studies have shown that black tea consumption may reduce cancer mortality, others have shown inconsistent effects. Findings have varied across demographics (e.g., sex, ethnicity) and type of cancer as well as tea type; thus, more research is needed. Results were strongest for a protective effect of green tea in oral cancer, consistent with other studies showing the beneficial antiviral, antibacterial, and antioxidant roles of catechins in oral health.

Many of the health effects from steeped green tea are found in doses higher than normally consumed, perhaps why **matcha**, a traditional Japanese powder made from finely ground green tea leaves, has gained favor in the US. (It is commonly added to water or milk to create a hot beverage far more concentrated than a steeped green tea; matcha can also be added to other foods for a nutrient and flavor boost.) There is likely little risk of overconsuming green tea when brewed, though flavonoids at very high doses, such as those found in dietary supplements (or, potentially, very high intakes of matcha), can have toxic effects. This is due to pro-oxidant effects—the opposite of its beneficial antioxidant effects at lower levels—that damage deoxyribonucleic acid (DNA) and cell membranes. Supplements (of any kind) can also be contaminated. Catechins in green tea may impair drug metabolism; those taking beta-blockers, lithium, estrogens, and other drugs or supplements should consult with a physician to be sure. Also, both black and white teas consumed in high doses have been found to impair iron metabolism and should be consumed with caution among those with iron deficiency anemia. And, like coffee, tea's caffeine content may be problematic for some, especially when consumed in excess. All of these effects are highly individual and dose-dependent, and the benefits of drinking tea far outweigh the potential risks for the majority.

15

ALCOHOL AND HEALTH

CHEERS!?

How is alcohol handled in the body?

Alcohol is among the only drugs consumed regularly in the diet other than caffeine. It is water-soluble and distributed into all tissues and fluids in relative proportion to water content. As a result, equal quantities of alcohol can produce a different blood alcohol concentration (BAC) based on lean and fat mass. Because women generally have a higher percentage of body fat compared to men, the distribution of alcohol throughout tissues is smaller, leading to a higher BAC for the same amount of alcohol.

Like other foodstuffs, alcohol passes through the alimentary tract into the stomach, and its movement into the small intestines is related to the rate of gastric emptying. It then moves across cell membranes to reach equilibrium as it is a toxin. Therefore, larger doses over short periods lead to a higher BAC compared to the same quantity consumed over a longer period. Gastric emptying, hence absorption, is faster when alcohol is consumed alone, the science behind the apt advice, "Don't drink on an empty stomach."

Alcohol is also a macronutrient, providing 7 calories/g compared to 9 in fat and 4 in both protein and carbs. Alcohol is not stored and must be metabolized and excreted and hence will be used for energy before any other nutrient. Thus, reducing alcohol consumption can be important in weight management in some individuals, particularly among heavy drinkers, since alcohol supplants the oxidation of other nutrients that will then be stored as fat unless otherwise compensated. Alcohol also suppresses vasopressin to some degree, the antidiuretic hormone allowing liquids to be absorbed rather than excreted, which is why drinking leads to urination, a diuretic effect. Even so, alcoholic drinks with high water content contribute to hydration, particularly when thirsty (which reflects underhydration). Indeed, diluted beer and wine were consumed regularly by people of all ages throughout human history for hydration as they were far safer to drink than unclean water.

The liver is the main site of alcohol metabolism, which is completed at the equivalent of 1 drink per hour on average, about 7 g/hour for a 70-kg individual. However, efficiency varies greatly due to metabolic rate as well as individual and genetic differences. "Alcohol flushing" is observed in some Asian subgroups, for example, due to polymorphisms that impede alcohol metabolism and cause the alcohol byproduct acetaldehyde to build up in the blood.

How do wine, beer, spirits, and cocktails differ in calorie and nutrient content?

In the US, drinks are defined according to alcohol content per "drink equivalent," which contains approximately 14 g of ethanol. Reference drinks are 12 fluid ounces of regular beer (5% alcohol), 5 fluid ounces of wine (12% alcohol), and 1.5 fluid ounces of 80-proof distilled spirit (40% alcohol). Alcohol concentration depends on fermentation (of all), proof (of spirits), and brew (of beer).

Where alcohol's impacts may vary depending on drink is at your waistline, a result of differing composition, hence calories. On average, a regular beer (12 ounces, 353 mL) is 153 calories, 91% water, and 13% carbs. "Light" beer is around 100 calories, a function of fewer carbs (~5%) and more water (94%). High-alcohol beer (like the double India pale ales [IPAs] I enjoy) can have 200 calories or more, with very few carbs (<1%) and 91% water. Because of its high water content, beer can contribute to hydration. Beer also contains small amounts of B-complex vitamins, phosphorus, potassium, calcium, silicon, and zinc, depending on its source grain.

Wine, like beer, varies in preparation, which in turn impacts its alcohol and water content. Sweeter wines have more carbohydrates (unsurprisingly), and all wines have potassium. The calorie content for a glass of wine, whether red, white, or rosé, is about 120 for a

5-ounce or 118-mL serving. Wine has less water (about 87%) and fewer carbs (3.8%) compared to beer. Red wine brings with it many phytochemicals, particularly polyphenols (Chapter 7), due to the inclusion of grape skins in its preparation. Liquor generally has the same amount of alcohol regardless of spirit and no carbohydrates: the differing calorie content results only from different alcohol percentage, or proof. Like beer and wine, higher alcohol content carries more calories and less water. For example, a 1.5-ounce shot (44 mL) of 80-proof vodka has 97 calories (67% water), 90-proof whiskey has 110 calories (62% water), and 100-proof tequila has 124 calories (58% water). Liquors have trace amounts of iron and zinc, while gin can include phytonutrients depending on its seasonings (e.g., juniper berries). Drink choice impacts energy content, obviously, first depending on how many shots of alcohol are included. A 1.5-ounce shot in a vodka-and-soda has a mere 97 calories but doubles with a double, logically. A pomegranate martini (another favorite of mine) can run more than 250 calories, depending on the specific mixers. And a luscious piñā colada in its usual hefty serving size can deliver more than 700 calories (!), including 94 g of sugar, or about 24 teaspoons.

What are the health risks and benefits of alcohol consumption?

Alcohol provides pleasure, like many other drugs, but is also highly addictive. Yet it also provides unique health benefits when consumed in moderate doses. Whether alcohol is protective or risky depends on drinking habits and genetic characteristics. Moderate intakes of alcohol, generally considered one daily drink (15 g of alcohol) for women and two drinks (30 g of alcohol) for men, are associated with a wide variety of positive health outcomes, including elevated high-density lipoprotein ("good") cholesterol (HDL), improved glucose metabolism and insulin sensitivity, less atherosclerosis and hypertension, reduced platelet aggregation, and decreased inflammation and blood clotting. These effects, likely in aggregate, convey a reduced risk of various diseases. The evidence is very strong that alcohol is protective for cardiovascular disease (CVD) in particular, a subject studied for decades. A 2011 systematic review and meta-analysis of 84 prospective studies, for instance, found reduced risks for CVD mortality (25%), coronary heart disease (39%), and all-cause mortality (23%) when comparing drinkers with nondrinkers; the lowest risk occurred with 2.5–14.9 g of alcohol daily. Many, many other reviews report similar protective results.

There is also substantial evidence that moderate alcohol consumers have a reduced risk of type 2 diabetes (T2DM) compared to abstainers. A meta-analysis of 38 studies revealed a protective effect with up to 63 g of alcohol daily—risk increased above this amount—with the greatest benefit at 10–14 g daily, yielding an 18% reduced risk. Interestingly, this study also showed that effects were relegated to women and non-Asian populations, unusual results that require replication. Decreased inflammation in the blood vessels of the brain, among other mechanisms, may contribute to a decreased risk of developing dementia, Alzheimer's, and Parkinson's—although a 2013 review found protective, adverse, or null effects of alcohol on risk of Alzheimer's, perhaps in part due to the complex and multifactorial nature of these diseases. More research is therefore needed.

Despite these benefits, alcohol can lead to a wide variety of problems throughout the digestive system, ranging from mild indigestion and acid reflux to a higher risk of some cancers. Chronic alcohol use gradually wears down the lining of the small intestine, impairing nutrient absorption and causing malnutrition and anemias in severe cases (like alcoholism). Normal blood sugar control can also be compromised. Alcohol impacts other organs and systems, too, from the skeletal (e.g., thinning bones) to the immune system (e.g., higher risk of infection). Over time, alcohol will destroy the liver: acute alcoholic hepatitis can lead to chronic liver inflammation and liver disease (cirrhosis). Cognitive impairment can also result from severe alcohol use. Many of these effects are caused by alcoholism, a physical dependency where systems and organs have been compromised and damaged and withdrawal can be fatal if unmanaged. Even so, heavy chronic drinking without alcoholism is a risk factor for hypertension, T2DM, heart disease, stroke, and overall increased morbidity and mortality and is responsible for toxic effects in many of the same organs protected at lower levels of consumption. And binge drinking—defined as 3–5 drinks in 2 hours and especially common in young adults—is associated with a higher risk of injuries and the development of alcohol use disorders.

Particularly dramatic is alcohol's clear relationship to an increased risk of breast cancer in women, a consistent finding thought to be due in part to alterations in hormones. Though originally the effect was seen mainly at intakes of alcohol greater than 2 drinks daily, newer research suggests an increased risk even among light drinkers. A recent review of 15 meta-analyses showed a dose–response relationship with breast cancer, estimating 144 000 cases and 38 000 deaths attributable to alcohol globally—and 18.8% of cases and 17.5% deaths were among light drinkers. Health-conscious women who enjoy alcohol consequently face a conundrum: moderate drinking is protective for heart health, although the same amount may increase risk of breast cancer; and heart disease is a much bigger killer of women than breast cancer.

The American Society of Clinical Oncology updated its statement on alcohol and cancer in 2018 on the basis of the current state of scientific evidence, including extensive reviews by the World Cancer Research Fund/American Institute for Cancer Research as well as the International Agency for Research on Cancer (IARC). There is also now consensus regarding alcohol's role in several other cancers beyond the breast. Evidence is "convincing" that alcohol is a cause of cancer of the oral cavity, pharynx, larynx, esophagus, liver, and colorectum (the latter of which is more consistent in men than women), even among moderate drinkers and perhaps, in the case of oral, esophageal, and breast cancers, light drinkers. Sites with direct alcohol exposure (i.e., larynx, esophagus, oral cavity/pharynx) among heavy drinkers carry the highest risk. Moreover, consuming higher amounts of alcohol from any source (wine, liquor, beer), over longer periods of time, increases risk, particularly for neck and head cancers. Based on these findings, alcohol is thus listed as a Group 1 carcinogen by the IARC, like tobacco.

Many of the above positive and negative effects reflect a J-shaped relationship, in which moderate drinkers have the greatest health benefits compared to abstainers or heavy drinkers; the poison, again, is in the dose. Still, variability in effects remains across cancer site (i.e., breast cancer risk may be linear) as well as age, sex, racial/ethnic group, and other factors. Newer research has discovered genetic factors that influence the harmful effect of alcohol on blood pressure, blood glucose, and triglycerides—and waist-to-hip ratio in South Korean men, for example, but not women. Importantly, there are salubrious diets like those of Seventh-day Adventists that are associated with longevity, less obesity, and lower disease that include little, if any, alcohol (Chapter 17).

If alcohol isn't already a part of your life, in moderation, experts agree that the potential risks from this addictive drug with its toxic effects are far too high to overcome its benefits.

Does red wine play a special role in heart disease prevention?

Wine became the focus of research during the last decade of the 20th century due to interest in the "French paradox" (coined in 1992), in which France enjoyed a lower prevalence of heart disease than the US and UK despite more smoking and higher saturated fat intake. Wine intake is higher in France than the US, particularly red wine, consumed in quantities of 20–30 g daily; and observational studies have shown about a 40% reduced risk of heart disease at these levels. Red wine is particularly high in a phytonutrient called resveratrol, a potent polyphenol antioxidant also found in grapes, peanuts, pomegranates, soybeans, raspberries, blueberries, apples, and plums. Grapes, wine, apples, peanuts, and soy are the major contributors to resveratrol in Western diets. But the highest concentrations are found in Japanese knotweed (*Polygonum japonicum*), which is used to make itadori tea, common in Japan and China.

Resveratrol has powerful effects when consumed in high doses in animal studies, particularly in reducing oxidative stress, and may be beneficial for reducing heart disease as well as other diseases, newer studies indicate. Consistently replicating results in humans has proved challenging, however, due to the difficulty in accurately assessing and isolating the effect of this singular component. Resveratrol's impact varies by how it's consumed, the presence of other dietary elements, chemical structure (there are numerous analogs that vary in bioactivity), and other factors. Furthermore, findings from clinical trials are inconsistent. It remains likely that resveratrol is beneficial for (heart) health, though the efficacious dose is currently estimated at 1 g daily, a quantity only accessible in pill form. To consume this quantity one would need to drink 505–2762 *liters* of red wine or eat 7143–33 333 *kilograms* of peanuts (!).

Research investigating potential differences between alcoholic drinks continues, including studies on resveratrol and wine in particular. For instance, a recent meta-analysis of 13 prospective studies with 397 296 individuals found the expected J-shaped relationship between alcohol and T2DM, but the strongest protective effects were seen at 20–30 g/day for wine and beer and 7–15 g/d for spirits, commensurate with a 20%, 9%, and 5% reduced risk, respectively. Though studies like this are interesting (and this one is strengthened by its inclusion of 13 reports), many observational investigations do not adequately control for other dietary and lifestyle factors; and wine drinkers are often different from beer and spirit drinkers in ways that may confound the relationship.

16

SWEET DRINKS

FRUIT JUICE, SUGAR-SWEETENED BEVERAGES, AND DIET SODA (POP)

How many sugar-sweetened beverages are we drinking, and are they related to obesity?

Beverages comprise 47% of added sugar intakes in American diets, of which 39% come from sugar-sweetened beverages (SSBs). SSBs include soft drinks (25%); fruit drinks, not including 100% fruit juices (11%); and sports and energy drinks (3%). A small percentage of SSBs come from coffee and tea, though the number is greater in places like the southeastern US, where "sweet tea" is a popular beverage. Added sugar content varies by drink, of course, from about 10 g in a light sports drink to about 50 g in an orange soda. Unsurprisingly, SSBs are strongly related to dental caries.

Calories from SSBs have risen dramatically in the US, from 95 calories daily in 1965 to 155 in 2010. In 2015, children and teenagers 4–18 years old consumed about 15–17 teaspoons of sugar daily on average, much of which came from SSBs. Intake varied across race/ethnicity and socioeconomic status, with black and Hispanic children consuming more SSBs than white children, particularly in lower-income families. SSBs, particularly soda pop, are also increasingly available in low- and middle-income countries—and remain a safer beverage to drink than unclean drinking water in some places.

The evidence base is considerable and convincing that SSBs contribute to weight gain and obesity in both children and adults, including results from a 2006 review of 30 investigations and a 2015 study analyzing 13 systematic literature reviews and meta-analyses. The effect is due in part to over-consumption of calories, a "lack of compensation" from liquid calories, in which the body seems less able to "compensate" for calories from liquids. In other words, calorie-laden beverages do not supplant other calorie-containing foods, they just add. As a result, people simply consume more calories overall when SSBs are included in the diet, thus facilitating a positive caloric balance that promotes weight gain.

The high glycemic index of SSBs leading to spikes in blood sugar and blood insulin can wear down insulin receptors, eventually leading to insulin resistance and type 2 diabetes mellitus (T2DM) in some people. A 2016 study examining 9 cohorts in aggregate saw a 26% increase in the risk of T2DM among SSB consumers, as well as a 28% increase in risk among sweetened fruit drink consumers. SSBs assessed in both longitudinal and intervention studies are also associated with higher blood pressure, blood lipids, and blood sugar, and other metabolic factors related to an increased risk of cardiovascular disease (CVD).

The strong evidence base and media firestorm surrounding soda and other SSBs in recent years has ignited a rash of public health and policy approaches designed to decrease consumption, particularly among children and teens. Some studies show decreased body weight when SSBs are replaced with water or other less caloric drinks or policies like soda taxes are employed to discourage consumption. Yet it's hard to imagine that anyone reading this book isn't aware that SSBs aren't the best choice for health, research notwithstanding, given that they are little more than sugar- and calorie-delivery vehicles with few, if any, nutrients.

Even so, emerging research suggests that some individuals are more likely to gain weight drinking SSBs than others, perhaps due to genetic differences. As well, rarely is a single component responsible for any disease or health outcome as diets are filled with myriad foods and drinks. In fact, SSBs have been around for more than a century, long before the epidemics of obesity, T2DM, and other chronic diseases took hold. Drinking SSBs infrequently, as a treat, is a fine choice as part of an otherwise healthy diet and lifestyle (Bourbon and ginger, anyone?). But when consumed in the amounts common among most Americans today, especially when part of a dietary pattern filled with other poor choices, they clearly aren't the best bet for optimal health and longevity.

While Americans have cut back on soda—per capita intake decreased 25% between 1998 and 2014 and has further declined since then—pop is taking a stronger hold elsewhere. Mexico consumes more soda than any other country per capita and has the highest rate of childhood obesity, for example, surpassing the US a few years back. Part of the soda habit is cultural: chubby kids represent adequate nourishment, as opposed to malnutrition, and soda has also been a historical go-to when water was unsafe. Mexico thus introduced a national soda tax that will hopefully translate to healthier waistlines, and early results appear promising. In the meantime, according to the 2016 report *Carbonating the World* from the US consumer advocacy organization Center for Science in the Public Interest, "Big Soda" is investing more than $40 billion in developing markets, targeting potential consumers in Africa, China, Indonesia, Brazil, India, and the Philippines— and still Mexico.

Is drinking fruit juice the same as eating whole fruit?

Fruit juice ranges in nutritional value depending on processing method and ingredients. Some retain much of the vitamins (like A and C), minerals, phytochemicals, and antioxidant activity of whole fruit, while others do not, though many lose their fiber. Fruit juices labeled "100% fruit" are the best choices, whereas "fruit drinks" can be comparable to soda in both sugar content and calories. For example, an 8-fluid-ounce (249 g) serving of 100% orange juice has 112 calories and 21 g of sugar, while the same serving of an orange fruit drink made with 5% juice has 120 calories and 29 g of sugar. An orange soda has 120 calories and 32 g of sugar. Only the 100% juice has calcium and protein. Both 100% juice and the fruit drink contain vitamin C, although the juice has 200% of one's daily requirement compared to only 70% in the drink (and none in the soda). Reading the nutrition facts panel and ingredients list is key.

The quick delivery of sugar and calories from juices is a disadvantage for regulating appetite and blood sugar. Research shows that liquids from any source do not register the same degree of fullness in the brain, often due to quicker consumption and gastric emptying. Consider the length of time it takes to drink a glass of orange juice versus eating an entire orange, for example, the latter of which requires chewing a fibrous solid. And this effect is also true for fruit drinks and 100% fruit juice, indeed any liquid: the body appears less able to register satiety and satiation compared to a solid. This means that drinking juices and other beverages that contain calories can lead to an overall higher energy intake. In other words, while energy intake from solid foods (like pizza) will register to the body as energy, eventually leading to feeling full, liquid foods (like fruit juice, soda, or beer) tend to pack on calories in a way the body doesn't recognize as quickly. This phenomenon is known as "caloric compensation" and helps people to regulate energy intake and maintain a healthy body weight. Therefore, because liquid foods don't have the same effect—they lack caloric compensation—they are more likely to put on extra pounds. Many studies have demonstrated that children have stronger caloric compensation than adults, perhaps because they are better able to recognize satiety cues. On the other hand, caloric compensation may be particularly poor in overweight individuals, who may already suffer from impaired satiety signals.

Is fruit juice a nutritious beverage or a risk factor for obesity, type 2 diabetes, and cavities? And is juicing healthy or hooey?

Although 100% fruit juice includes calories and (natural, not added) sugars, there are copious studies showing that it can contribute to an overall healthy dietary pattern, likely because it has been a hallmark of healthy diets for decades and remains correlated with other healthy behaviors in many population subgroups (think a glass of orange juice with breakfast).

Fruit juice may be especially beneficial for children. A 2015 study found that consumption of fruit juice at the levels recommended by the American Pediatric Association helps children meet nutritional needs, especially for vitamin C and potassium (and other phytonutrients, depending on the juice and production method). Another extensive review of studies between 1995 and 2013 found that the majority did not see an association between fruit juice consumption and obesity. Some also showed that children drinking 100% fruit juice had higher intakes of fiber, vitamin C, magnesium, and potassium, without contributing to obesity. A 2017 review confirmed these findings in children as well as adults.

Still, fruit juice (and other beverages with sugar) remains an established risk factor for dental caries at high intakes, and some fruit juices containing fructose and sorbitol (a sugar alcohol) can lead to diarrhea in toddlers. For these and other reasons, the American Academy of Pediatrics 2017 guideline recommends that children under 1 year should not drink fruit juice at all and that intake should be limited to 4 ounces daily (about half the daily fruit recommendation) for infants. Consistent with the evidence, the guidelines also indicate that while excessive fruit juice consumption can lead to gastrointestinal distress in children and weight gain, fruit juice can nonetheless be part of a healthy and balanced diet. And it can be particularly economical in providing valuable nutrients and phytochemicals to low-income families to help them meet their fruit needs.

"Juicing" has become trendy among health and fitness enthusiasts, a quick way to deliver calories, vitamins, and phytonutrients in creative concoctions pleasing to the eye as well as the palate. Many home-juicing systems eliminate or reduce the fiber compared to the whole fruit, though blending can ameliorate this effect. But even fresh juice can provide the same quick boost of energy and spikes in blood sugar and insulin as any other 100% fruit juice, depending on ingredients—and the same issues related to lack of caloric compensation pertain. It also takes a lot of volume and produce (and special equipment, often) to build just one glass, making it generally far more expensive than whole fruit.

A fascinating 2017 study found that juice was an incredibly rich source of antioxidants that can deliver an immediate boost to some tissues. Results varied, however, by the type of juice (i.e., which vegetables and fruits were included) and the amount and frequency of consumption. An individual's baseline health, weight, sex, age, and genetics also mattered, as did overall diet and exercise patterns. Thus, juice may be part of salubrious diet for some, but it is certainly not a health elixir. And whole fruit is generally more satiating, has fewer calories, is less expensive, is better calorically compensated, and creates less food waste.

Are diet beverages helpful for weight control?

Given that much of the problem with SSBs is due to sugar, it is reasonable to wonder whether beverages made with low-calorie or non-nutritive sweeteners (LCS or NNS, respectively, referred to collectively as "diet" beverages herein) are useful alternatives for calorie control and weight loss. To date, scientific evidence on whether diet SSBs are helpful—or even harmful—for weight loss and weight control is inconsistent. Are those drinking diet SSBs doing so as part of an unhealthful diet, the "potato chips and diet Coke" stereotype? Or are consumers choosing diet SSBs to help cut back on sugar and calories as part of an otherwise nutritious diet and healthy lifestyle? And are effects on appetite, weight, and health positive or negative?

A decade of research conducted mostly in animal models suggests that "the uncoupling of sweet taste and caloric intake by low-calorie sweeteners (LCS) can disrupt an animal's ability to predict the metabolic consequences of sweet taste, and thereby impair the animal's ability to respond appropriately to sweet-tasting foods." Specifically, animals with long-term, chronic exposure to LCS (including sucralose, saccharin, acesulfame potassium, aspartame, or the combination of erythritol and aspartame) actually *gain* weight due to lower energy expenditure and overconsumption of sweet and fatty foods. Some animals also showed increased blood glucose and insulin compared to animals drinking water or, surprisingly, even full-calorie counterparts. Results vary, however; and ill effects are especially pronounced among animals with a genetic predisposition to obesity and those consuming a typical Western diet.

Even so, findings in some animal models are in tandem with a few prospective observational studies that, counterintuitively, show that diet SSBs *increased* the risk of obesity and cardiometabolic disease—though others show no effect. Reverse causality is possible even in longitudinal studies, in which those consuming more diet soda are perhaps trying to lose weight but are unsuccessful; hence, increased consumption is then correlated with higher weight. Lack of adjustment for potential confounders—like other dietary behaviors and health behaviors—may also contribute to unexpected findings.

Thus, while the verdict is still out on whether LCS or NNS are ultimately helpful or harmful—physiological effects related to satiety signals, taste perception, and appetite remain under investigation—a number of studies in humans indicate that diet SSB drinkers have healthier habits than nonconsumers on average. One study, for instance, indicated that 19.5% of American adults consumed diet SSBs and that intakes were not related to weight or health. Consumers also had a higher overall diet score, less smoking, and more physical activity, suggesting that diet SSBs were part of a nexus of healthy behaviors.

The inconsistent observational evidence on diet SSBs spurred a number of randomized controlled trials (RCTs) in the past several years, and a 2014 meta-analysis shed additional light on the relationship. Though the study included LCS from food as well as beverages, the 15 RCTs showed that LCS foodstuffs were associated with lower body weight, body mass index (BMI), fat mass, and waist circumference; the 9 prospective cohort studies showed no relation to body weight and fat mass. Together, the results suggest that diet SSBs may help modestly with weight loss when substituted for full-calorie versions.

Because the RCTs differed in the substitution beverage, however, additional studies investigated whether diet beverages and water had similar effects on weight loss and weight maintenance. A 2016 RCT tested whether 24 ounces (710 mL) of water versus the same amount of NNS beverages among 303 weight-stable participants in a weight loss program impacted subsequent weight and cardiometabolic risk factors over a 1-year study period. Those receiving NNS beverages maintained a significantly larger weight loss compared to those consuming water (6.21 versus 2.45 kg). NNS drinkers also lost significantly more waist circumference. Interestingly, the water consumers reported feeling hungrier following the intervention, while the NNS drinkers reported no difference in hunger. These results need further replication, and new trials are underway to better understand whether diet SSBs are consistently related to better health outcomes compared to water (or other unsweetened beverages, even, like coffee or tea).

Weight loss by any reasonable means is paramount given the escalated risks attributed to excess body fat, Thus, studies showing overall positive impacts for diet SSBs are helpful in light of the obesity and chronic disease epidemics. Still, choosing beverages like unsweetened coffee or tea rather than SSBs will decrease calories and added sugar while helping retrain palates to prefer less sweet foods—and provide a health boost not available from diet SSBs, too. (Herbal iced tea is my go-to.)

Part V

DIETS FOR OPTIMAL HEALTH, LONGEVITY, AND SUSTAINABILITY

TODAY AND TOMORROW

When it comes to diet, the whole is greater than the sum of its parts—and one size doesn't fit all. Mountains of information have accumulated over time and space, culture and place, to inspire a health-giving, planet-saving diet. And evidence-based data from the social sciences illuminates strategies for creating long-lasting dietary changes. How will evolutions in science and developments in technology dovetail with changes in consumer lifestyles and preferences to create the future of food? And how can we ensure that tomorrow's world is healthier and more sustainable for ourselves and our planet?

17

PUTTING IT ALL TOGETHER

CREATING A HEALTH-GIVING DIET THAT WORKS FOR YOU, FOR LIFE

Is focusing on individual nutrients and foods important for health?

Nutrition is a biomedical science with roots in analytical chemistry. As such, it has relied traditionally upon reductionism, the philosophy dominating traditional Western medicine that reduces phenomena to their smallest components. In the case of nutrition, this means individual nutrients or foods are often examined to elucidate diet–disease relationships. While such "single-nutrient" (and "single-food") investigations are necessary, particularly when establishing biological mechanisms responsible for cause and effect, they are limited in the questions they can answer. Moreover, observational studies focused on single elements may be biased by unaccounted dietary variables. Randomized controlled trials (RCTs) overcome some methodological challenges through randomization and control groups but can still be plagued by reductionist thinking. Single-nutrient studies are further restricted in how helpful they are to individual eaters seeking practical diet advice, who can't reasonably track each individual element (e.g., grams of fat) important for health, or in what amounts.

These limitations and others gradually led to a call from nutrition scientists to focus on the whole diet—that is, the usual foods and drinks that, together, characterize how and what you eat. "Dietary patterns" not only better reflect actual eating behavior but account for nutrient synergies in the body and intercorrelations: those who consume breakfast cereal, for instance, also likely consume milk and fruit and a cup of coffee, together in the same meal, impacting digestion and absorption. These food and meal combinations, and everything else consumed throughout the day, week, and year, are what really matter, a truism now supported by a plethora of research.

In turn, many countries and organizations today are creating dietary guidelines based on overarching principles that reflect the whole diet rather than individual components. This is not to say that recommendations on specific food groups or nutrients aren't important, however. Increasing servings of vegetables and fruits is a central dietary goal, for instance, informed by "single food (group)" studies. Likewise, the Dietary Reference Intakes (DRIs) in the US and Canada (formerly known as the Recommended Dietary Allowances, or RDAs) provide nutrient-based guidelines and policies that ensure adequate and safe intakes that prevent deficiency and toxicity, both of which can be fatal.

The upshot? Don't lose the forest for the trees: your overall dietary pattern—not any single nutrient or food, even those flaunted as a "superfood"—is the most powerful contributor to health, wellbeing, and disease. The dietary gestalt—the whole is greater than the sum of its individual parts—is as true for what we eat as it is for anything else.

Are there universal dietary principles for preventing chronic disease?

Dietary advice comes in a number of forms, including recommended intakes of specific nutrients and food-based guidelines, which are updated as nutrition knowledge evolves. The World Health Organization (WHO) helps member nations develop country-specific guidelines to reduce the burden of chronic disease through its five dietary principles: (1) Achieve a healthy weight through energy balance; (2) Increase plant-based foods like vegetables and fruits, legumes, whole grains, and nuts; (3) Limit added sugar intake; (4) Limit salt intake and ensure that salt is iodized; and (5) Limit total fat intake, shift from saturated toward unsaturated fats, and eliminate trans fats, WHO further notes that "[i]mproving dietary habits is a societal, not just an individual problem" and "demands a population-based, multisectoral, multi-disciplinary, and culturally relevant approach."

Individual countries create their own national dietary guidelines to direct citizens toward better health by focusing on commonly consumed foods that address key nutrition problems. Recommendations are generally used to direct federal nutrition and food policies, programs, and educational initiatives but are also adapted for public use. State and local organizations and institutions then customize guidelines to meet the specific needs of their populations.

There is remarkable consistency among the core dietary guidelines of most countries, the majority of which emphasize such elements as consuming a variety of foods; balancing energy intake to maintain a healthy weight; limiting saturated fat, sugar, and sodium; and increasing plant foods, particularly vegetables and fruits. Whole grains, beans and legumes, and dairy are also encouraged. The Dietary Guidelines for Americans, for example, emphasizes the total eating pattern in its "MyPlate" infographic, which includes a plate and a "dairy" cup/bowl. The guidelines highlight that "recommendations for healthy eating patterns should be applied in their entirety, given the interconnected relationship that each dietary component can have with each other." The UK Eatwell Guide provides similar advice in a pie chart and specifies that "[y]ou don't need to achieve this balance with every meal but try to get the balance right over a day or even a week." A cup of water also appears as part of its graphic, and individuals are encouraged to consult food labels when making dietary choices.

India's guidelines accentuate similar food groups and dietary principles to those in the US and UK and are presented graphically in its food pyramid. However, its core recommendations include 15 principles that address the needs of vulnerable populations; nutritional needs during growth and development; child and elder malnutrition; women's health, pregnancy, and breastfeeding; and food security and safety. This difference is because India must focus on food security and safety and maternal and child mortality, still major public health problems, in addition to addressing the growing burden of chronic diseases.

Some variability nonetheless remains in how policymakers and educators interpret science and communicate it to the public.

Highlighting areas of particular need in a society is paramount, though food, agriculture, and economic politics may also play a role. There are also a few legitimate places in nutrition where scientists reach different conclusions on the available data, as in any field. One example is Harvard's Healthy Eating Plate, which has many similarities and a few notable differences compared to USDA's MyPlate. It discourages potatoes and refined grains (although evidence from total diet research shows that these foods can play a role in a healthy diet, in moderation). As well, the plate does not emphasize total fat, the way that the guidelines from WHO and many other groups do. This is largely due to substantial scientific evidence from Mediterranean diets, which are higher in total fat due to the intake of olive oil yet are protective for heart disease. Indeed, the vast scientific consensus is that unsaturated fats are healthier than solid fats, though there is considerable research that limiting total fat can be important for some people, particularly in weight control. Even so, experts agree that one size doesn't fit all: health-giving diets can vary in fat content assuming that they promote a healthy weight and embrace variety, balance, and moderation across all foods and drinks. And the broad consensus is that creating a plant-based diet rich in vegetables, fruits, whole grains, lean proteins, and healthy oils that limits sugar and salt is key.

Is a calorie just a calorie? What mix of fat, carbs, and protein is most effective for weight management?

The vilification of fat in the US stimulated the low-fat/high-carb craze of the 1980s and 90s, yet during this time the nation also got heavier. Other countries soon gained weight, creating an obesity pandemic tied directly to the growing burden of chronic diseases worldwide (Chapter 2). Correlation does not equal causation, however: many other diet and lifestyle changes have occurred in the US and other Western countries since the onset of the epidemic. Eating away from home and portion sizes increased in the late 20th century (Chapter 5) alongside sedentary activity, while physical activity and smoking have decreased. These and other factors are likely contributors to the obesity epidemic.

Diet nevertheless plays a key role. But is a calorie just a calorie when it comes to weight, or does diet composition matter? This question has been a major research focus for the past several decades. And the obvious temporal association between the onset of low-fat diets and the escalation of obesity led some to question whether fat is really all that. An initial spotlight on high-protein diets (Chapter 8) has burgeoned into a large body of literature comparing how equal-calorie (i.e., isoenergetic) diets with varying proportions of fats, protein, and carbohydrate—for example, medium-fat/low-protein/high-carb, medium-fat/medium-protein/medium-carb, high-fat/high-protein/low-carb, and the like—impact weight loss.

While findings from individual studies vary somewhat, results in aggregate show little, if any, significant differences in weight loss across diets of varying compositions in well-designed studies with follow-up of at least 1 or 2 years. For example, a 2015 meta-analysis of 19 RCTs found that weight loss was not different comparing those following a low-fat or a moderate-fat diet. In other studies, similar weight loss was also observed comparing high-protein to low-fat diets or low-carbohydrate to high-carbohydrate diets. One interesting trial showed that, in addition to comparable weight loss after 2 years, satiety, hunger, and satisfaction were similar. Only higher session attendance was associated with more weight loss, an indicator of commitment and adherence to the diet.

A few specific types of diets at the extreme ranges of carbohydrate intake are noteworthy. Low- and very low-carb ketogenic diets (i.e., ones that burn fat for energy rather than carbohydrate and produce ketone byproducts detectable in urine) yield more weight loss and greater favorable effects on cardiometabolic risk factors compared to low-fat diets (<30% of energy). While critical for some people—ketogenic diets are used to effectively control seizures in epilepsy—very low-carb diets (<50 grams daily) are hard for many people to follow long term as they greatly constrain (luscious) staple foods like bread, pasta, and vegetables.

Very high-carb vegetarian diets are at the other end of the spectrum. A meta-analysis of 12 RCTs observed greater weight loss among vegetarians compared to omnivores. Differences dissipated after 1 year, however, consistent with other studies showing attenuated effects with longer follow-up. While vegetarians also tend to have other positive lifestyle habits, a sizable body of observational studies shows that vegetarians consuming diets high in fiber-rich foods like vegetables, beans, and whole grains tend to be leaner and have less body fat compared to omnivores. Studies like these underscore the fundamental nutrition principle that it's the source and type of carb—and fat, and protein—that's key, not the quantity.

Part of the weight loss picture is whether factors like biological sex, clinical status, or genetics interact with diet. A systematic review found that men lost more weight than women on average, whatever diet they followed—a frustrating fact many women already realize anecdotally—though differences were small. Weight loss may also vary by health condition. One study randomly assigned overweight individuals with type 2 diabetes mellitus (T2DM) to a medium-fat diet that was either high-protein/medium-carb or low-protein/high-carb. Both groups attended 18 sessions over 12 months, and weight loss and waist circumference changes were similar at the 2-year follow-up. Notably, there was very little difference in actual protein intake between groups at the end of the study, again illustrating the difficulty in long-term adherence to high-protein diets for many.

While more will continue to be learned about how different groups respond to different weight loss diets, what is clear is that many approaches can yield positive results. In many ways, therefore, a calorie is just a calorie: excess intake relative to expenditure (positive caloric balance) leads to weight gain. Despite findings that some diets perform better than others in individual studies, perhaps due in part to unmeasured food and dietary preferences that impact long-term participation, short follow-up, or genetic differences, the majority of research indicates that a specific macronutrient composition is less important than adherence: sticking to whatever plan that fosters a negative caloric balance is key.

That said, diet composition *is* helpful as a function of the varied metabolic effects of macronutrients on metabolism (Chapter 8). Controlling appetite without feeling deprived is critical, which is why protein and fat are helpful due to their greater satiety and satiation that promote fullness compared to carbs, for instance, helping to restrain calorie intake. An additional body of research suggests that consuming high-volume foodstuffs low in energy density, such as fiber- and water-rich foods like vegetables and soups, can also create fullness on fewer calories. Impacts on cardiovascular risk factors like high-density lipoprotein ("good") and low-density lipoprotein ("bad") cholesterol (HDL and LDL, respectively), fasting glucose and insulin, and the like also differ by macronutrient composition: a calorie is *not* just a calorie given the unique biochemistry of fats, carbs, and proteins. Overall metabolic and clinical profiles are important, too: one study observed that those with T2DM or prediabetes had more favorable insulin and lipid responses following a Mediterranean or moderate-fat diet rather than a high-carb/low-fat diet—particularly if those carbs come from refined grain foods that have a negative impact on blood sugar and insulin (Chapter 10). However weight is lost, keeping off pounds is paramount. A number of studies support the beneficial effect of daily physical activity, social support, pharmaceuticals, acupuncture, commercial weight loss plans, grocery lists, and problem-solving therapy, some of which have a genetic basis, just like diet itself. For example, the Diet, Obesity and Genes trial among 932 European families compared weight maintenance among 5 ad libitum (non-calorie-restricted/eating at will) diets that varied protein intake and glycemic index (GI, Chapter 8) while keeping the same fat intake. Those consuming a higher-protein/lower-GI diet kept the most weight off, a result found in other studies. The effectiveness of such a diet may be a result of genetic variability. Another study found that protein was especially beneficial for weight loss among those with a certain allele of the obesity-associated *FTO* gene. In time, more studies like these will elucidate what weight loss diets, and which behavioral strategies, are most successful, and in which individuals, as we inch slowly toward personalized nutrition (Chapter 18).

What popular diets are best for weight loss?

Fad and celebrity diets and legitimate commercial weight loss plans have always been around to provide eaters dieting options, each touted as *the best*. But is there really only one way to lose weight? Is one program truly superior? The basis for efficacy of popular weight loss diets harkens back to biochemistry: the different effects of fat, carbs, and protein on appetite, food intake, and energy expenditure are key (Chapter 8). Diets also differ not just in their composition but in other factors too, including such things as social support, portion control, and food provision.

While many individual studies evoke provocative headlines, an example of "single-study sensationalism," many are biased due to inadequate follow-up: short-term weight loss is often different compared to results obtained over 1 year or more. A 2015 Cochrane review comparing Weight Watchers, Jenny Craig, Nutrisystem, Medifast, Optifast, Atkins, and SlimFast, for example, found that weight loss differences initially observed dissipated over a longer follow-up. Similar findings were seen in a rigorous review of 12 RCTs comparing Atkins, South Beach, Weight Watchers, and Zone diets, showing that all participants lost weight. And yet another meta-analysis of 48 RCTs found similar results comparing a wide range of popular low-fat and low-carb diets, including Atkins, Weight Watchers, Ornish, and the Zone—as well as the Biggest Loser, Jenny Craig, Nutrisystem, and Volumetrics. As importantly, many of these studies demonstrated that whatever diet followed led to significantly greater weight loss compared to the control group receiving only diet education, "usual care" (e.g., exercise, attitudes, nutrition), or generic nutrition counseling.

Professional organizations like the American Heart Association, the American College of Cardiology, and The Obesity Society concur: weight loss is similar across popular diets, and current scientific evidence is inadequate to recommend one plan over another.

The upshot? Having *some* kind of plan is important, and following one that works *for you* is critical: study after study shows that adherence is what leads to weight loss, not the dietary particulars. (A clever nutrition professor made this point by following the "Twinkie diet", losing 27 pounds in 10 weeks—though, to be clear, he also ate Oreos, Doritos, and powdered donuts. That said, don't do that.)

Do calorie restriction and fasting lead to a longer life and better health?

A calorie is the unit of energy (heat) needed to raise 1 gram of water 1°C. (A joule is the international scientific unit, equal to 0.239 calories.) This is why nutrition scientists and others often use "calorie" and "energy" interchangeably. The calorie counts of food are technically kilocalories, or 1000 "small" calories (e.g., an 80-"calorie" apple is actually 80 kilocalories, or 80 000 calories). The measurement of calories is quite difficult to quantify with complete accuracy. Even so, considering calories is important to some degree, particularly relatively speaking. In other words, whatever error surrounds measuring precisely the amount of calories in an orange versus ice cream is nevertheless informative in demonstrating that the ice cream is far more energy-dense.

All animals, including our own species, tend to consume the amount of calories they require to maintain a stable weight based on metabolic needs, age, sex, and physical activity; this is why weight doesn't fluctuate when energy expenditure and energy intake are stable. How many total calories we ingest and expend (i.e., caloric balance) shapes body weight, and diet composition critically influences disease risk and health. At the same time, total calories consumed relative to biological needs plays a paramount role in longevity, regardless of source. Indeed, one of the best-supported but little-known facts in nutrition is that caloric restriction (CR) increases life span and delays the onset of and reduces the risk for many chronic diseases of aging across many species.

The hypothesis that reducing calories while still meeting nutrient needs prolonged life was first tested in rodents in 1935. Studies have since been replicated in hundreds of animal models, and epidemiologic observations have also suggested that those on naturally lower-calorie diets, including some vegetarian and vegan populations, have greater longevity and less chronic disease. While precise mechanisms remain undiscovered, there are myriad pathways by which CR alters metabolism, metabolic functioning (like insulin sensitivity and inflammation responses), and neuroendocrine processes that, doubtless synergistically, increase life span.

The 1990s Biosphere 2 project, designed to study human life within a self-contained ecosystem, was the first inadvertent "experiment" in CR, a result of unanticipated scarce food production. Diets were high in nutrients yet low in energy, resulting in decreased blood sugar, cholesterol, triglycerides, blood pressure, and body weight. The Caloric Restriction Society International was founded in 1994 (by Biosphere's chief medical officer and others) as a resource and support for CR enthusiasts who reduce calories between 10% and 40% to foster longevity.

The first RCT studying CR in nonobese people occurred in 2006, with participants split into 3 groups: 25% CR, 12.5% CR plus a 12.5% increase in exercise, and a very-low-calorie (890 kilocalories/day) diet until 15% weight reduction, followed by weight maintenance. After 6 months, the metabolism of each of the groups increased compared to the control group—significantly more than expected as a function of weight loss—including lower fasting insulin and body temperature. They also showed reduced oxygen consumption, resulting in fewer reactive oxygen species and less deoxyribonucleic acid (DNA) damage, both of which are related to aging and disease.

The findings of this small trial stimulated a larger research effort, resulting in the CALERIE (Comprehensive Assessment of Long-term Effects of Reducing Intake of Energy) consortium. This RCT studied 218 nonobese participants assigned either to a 25% CR or to an ad libitum (i.e., nonrestrictive) control diet over the course of 2 years, finding beneficial effects on body weight, body composition, and cardiometabolic risk factors that were sustained 2 years following the end of the study. Numerous peer-reviewed reports have been published from the CALERIE group, showing that CR is safe and effective and does not lead to negative consequences (e.g., poor mood, sleep, or sexual functioning). A recent 2017 investigation also found that CR reduced the rate of biological aging among participants. While the impact on longevity itself cannot be ascertained in the CALERIE study for some years, if ever—such studies are infeasible—the data thus far are consistent with scientific evidence in other species showing that CR increases life span.

Despite these robust findings, nutrition professionals do not generally emphasize CR as a health strategy. There are many reasons, including the possibility of inducing eating-disordered behavior in those susceptible. As well, the amount of CR needed to achieve desired results is substantial—you will be hungry, often—and thus its appeal to the general population is limited. As a result, a number of scientists are seeking to create a mimetic, a "have your cake and eat it too," approach that imitates the effects of CR on longevity without actually having to reduce calories. Interestingly, some studies suggest that resveratrol (Chapter 15), the bioactive phytochemical found in red wine and other foods, may mimic the effects of CR through its impact on sirtuins, molecules that influence energy metabolism and insulin response through their role in gene transcription and DNA repair. (One company is already testing such a drug.) Whether a CR mimetic will provide access to the ever-elusive fountain of youth remains to be seen. Thus, some "longevity scientists" strive to increase healthful life span without succumbing to the chronic diseases of aging followed by a quick, painless death, a concept known as "compressed morbidity."

Achieving longer life requires slowing aging significantly, however, not just preventing disease. In fact, some believe it is possible to delay death for quite some time, possibly indefinitely, in which the next significant advance will blend cutting-edge science and engineering innovations of today, or tomorrow. Ideas include growing new organs using genetic engineering; hacking longevity genes and editing out aging; manipulating the epigenome (chemical components that affect how DNA translates its instructions, thereby modifying its function); creating optimally nutrified food suited to an individual's specific genome; or manufacturing a "god" pill. Futurist Ray Kurzweil predicts *Homo sapiens* will merge with artificial intelligence via robotics or the cloud and employ nanobots to scour the blood and remove anti-aging elements. However it's done, technologies informed by genetics, big data, high tech, and machine learning will doubtless be involved in increasing longevity in some capacity. (Engineers and scientists at Google are already working on it, as are others.)

While extreme longevity and (potential) immortality are a while away, CR remains the only current known method of increasing life span. A related concept gaining research (and media) attention is fasting. Fasting has long been a part of many religious traditions as a form of penance and spiritual growth and has also been used in some ancient healing practices. In recent years, fasting has become a popular way to control weight and improve health and longevity, perhaps as it's more appealing than severely cutting calories.

There are varying forms fasting can take, including periodic prolonged fasting (e.g., 2 or more consecutive days), intermittent fasting (e.g., 1–2 days fasting, 5–6 days regular eating), time-restricted fasting (e.g., prolonging the fast following sleep and restricting food intake to only 8 hours daily), and alternate-day fasting. One exciting study showed that prolonged fasting changes cellular activity and ultimately promotes stress resistance, renewal, and regeneration of stem cells in particular; multiple cycles of fasting even abate immunosuppression and mortality caused by chemotherapy in mice, also observed in preliminary data in a few human cancer patients. Other animal studies show that, similar to CR, prolonged fasting not only leads to prevention or delayed onset of diseases but may also help to reverse extant disease. Another study in mice, also piloted in a very small group of humans, showed that following a very low-calorie, low-protein diet that mimics fasting for 5 days per month followed by regular eating the remaining days led to favorable biomarkers of organ and system regeneration consistent with longevity.

Studies like these are titillating but require far more research with more (human) participants and longer follow-up. In one small experiment, a 1-day water-only fast among 30 people showed differences in biomarkers like hemoglobin, human growth hormone, red blood cell count, hematocrit, and HDL cholesterol and decreased triglycerides and weight. Most returned to baseline levels 48 hours after the fast, except for weight and triglycerides. Numerous other small studies, including RCTs, show beneficial effects of prolonged fasting on similar disease biomarkers.

The study of intermittent fasting (IF) has been conducted most often in comparison to other forms of CR as a weight loss strategy. A 2015 review identified only 6 small studies, showing that IF resulted in similar weight loss compared to continuous CR. One study showed a greater body fat loss in IF, however; and 2 showed bigger decreases in insulin resistance. Another study comparing IF with continuous CR showed similar effects among those with T2DM. In addition, a number of studies among those observing Ramadan, a month-long period in which many Muslims fast from dusk to dawn, demonstrated beneficial effects on blood glucose, insulin, and insulin resistance among normal-weight individuals in addition to mild weight loss. All studies were small and of short duration (<6 months), thus warranting much longer and larger investigations.

It also seems likely that different types of fasting evoke diverse metabolic effects, whether in animals or in humans. For example, a 2014 review of 59 animal studies comparing CR, ketogenic diets, and IF on cancer found that both CR and ketogenic diets showed anticancer effects but IF did not. Yet other reviews concluded that both prolonged fasting and IF have protective effects on a wide range of conditions in animal studies, similar to CR, and included not only cancer but also neurological disorders like Alzheimer's and Parkinson's diseases and stroke.

Time-restricted fasting (TRF) is a type of IF based on the intersection of sleep and feeding cycles by extending the natural fast following sleep to 12 or more hours, thus limiting eating time. TRF experiments in animals show robust results on glucose and lipid biomarkers, though data are scarce in humans. Newer studies are unraveling the degree to which protein (and specific amino acids) intake and the microbiome (Chapter 4) work in concert with circadian rhythms to promote longevity.

Current findings are promising but many research gaps remain, highlighting the need for more studies given the potential impact of fasting in its various forms on chronic disease prevention, treatment, and longevity.

What are the keys to longevity? What are the "Blue Zones"?

While science and technology may one day solve the pesky problems of aging and death, today we are left with low-tech solutions to enhance health and longevity by following the fundamental dietary principles discussed herein. Individuals must nonetheless put everything together in a way that works for them, which can differ widely depending on such factors as tradition and culture, palate, and lifestyle. The Blue Zones—populations where longevity is pronounced as measured by the high proportion of centenarians relative to average rates—provide valuable insights on the similarities and differences of five regions where people thrive.

The "Blue Zone" concept was coined by demographer Michel Poulain in 2000 to characterize groups that lived longer, suffered from fewer (if any) chronic diseases, and had greater physical and mental agility compared to the general population. Poulain and colleagues described the first Blue Zone in a 2004 study, showing that the Ogliastra region of Sardinia, Italy, had the highest percentage of centenarian men in the world. Four more Blue Zones were later discovered. One thousand miles south of Tokyo, Okinawa, Japan, boasts the highest number of centenarian women; Latin Americans in the Nicoya Peninsula of Costa Rica have the second highest concentration of male centenarians and the lowest rate of middle-age mortality; Ikaria, Greece, enjoys the world's lowest rates of dementia and one of the lowest rates of middle-age mortality; and Seventh-day Adventists in the Loma Linda region of California live more than 10 years longer on average compared to other Americans.

Despite shared longevity and healthful aging, there are notable dietary differences across regions (Table 17.1). There is little to no overlap in key foods consumed, which reflects the indigenous crops and livestock across diverse topography and geography that have shaped culinary traditions. Grass-fed dairy, usually from sheep or goats, is a part of some diets, reflecting traditional agriculture and pastoral lifestyles. Fish is a small component of the Okinawan and Ikarian coastal diets but not the others. Only Loma Lindans are largely vegetarian, due to religious beliefs; they have the lowest consumption of animal foods. Coffee, tea, and water are the major beverages consumed throughout the Blue Zones. Alcohol contributes moderately in the Mediterranean and minimally in the Okinawan diets—and little, if at all, in the Loma Lindan population. The two Mediterranean diets are closest in composition, unsurprisingly: both feature olive oil, bread, legumes, and cheese. Yet the Sardinian diet includes far more carbohydrates, dairy, and alcohol as the region is highly mountainous: herding sheep is common, as is growing grapes. In contrast, the Ikarian diet has a much higher fat content and a larger variety of vegetables and fruits from its fertile farmland.

At the same time, health-giving, disease-fighting food groups identified throughout this book—vegetables and fruits; coffee, tea, and water; beans and legumes; whole grains—are common across the Blue Zones. Meat of any kind is eaten in small amounts, if at all, and usually reserved for special occasions—and it is not processed using methods that add sodium, nitrates, and other ingredients.

Table 17.1 Diet Composition, Food, and Beverage Intakes Across the 5 Blue Zones

Blue Zone	Diet Composition (Highest to Lowest as a Percentage of Daily Calories)	Common Foods & Drinks
Sardinia, Italy	Grains: 47% Dairy: 26% Vegetables: 12% Meat, fish, poultry: 5% Legumes: 4% Sugars: 3% Added fats: 2%	Barley, fava beans, chickpeas, tomatoes, fennel, whole wheat sourdough bread, almonds, milk (goat or sheep), dairy, particularly pecorino cheese; cannonau grenache wine (3–4 small [3–4 ounces] glasses daily)
Okinawa, Japan	Sweet potatoes: 67% Rice: 12% Other vegetables: 9% Legumes: 6% Other grains: 3% Fish, meat, poultry: 2% Other foods: 1%	*Imo* purple or yellow sweet potatoes, brown rice, tofu, bitter melon (goya), seaweeds (especially kombu and wakame), shiitake mushrooms, pork, garlic, turmeric; green jasmine tea, locally brewed *awamori* (millet brandy), sake
Ikaria, Greece	Other vegetables: 20% Greens: 17% Fruits: 16% Legumes: 11% Potatoes: 9% Olive oil: 6% Fish: 6% Pasta: 5% Meat: 5% Sweets 4%	Olive oil, wild greens and herbs, potatoes, goat's milk feta cheese, black-eyed peas, chickpeas, lemons, honey; coffee, herbal tea, red wine
Nicoya Peninsula, Costa Rica	Grains: 26% Dairy: 24% Vegetables: 14% Added sugars: 11% Fruits: 9% Legumes: 7% Meat, fish, poultry: 5% Nuts and seeds: 2% Added fats: 2% Eggs: 2%	Maize *nixtamal* (corn tortillas), squash, black beans ("3 sisters"), rice, yams, papaya, banana, peach palms (*pejivalles*); water
Loma Linda, US	Vegetables: 33% Fruits: 27% Legumes and soy: 12% Dairy: 10% Grains: 7% Meat and poultry: 4% Nuts and seeds: 2% Added fats: 2% Fish: 1% Eggs: 1% Added sugars: 1%	Avocado, beans, nuts, oatmeal, whole wheat bread, soy milk, salmon; water (at least 6 glasses daily); alcohol is not permitted, though some do drink

Data are summarized from *Blue Zones: The Science of Living Longer* (Washington, DC: National Geographic Partners, 2016).

Very little sugar and salt is consumed, a reflection in part of the lack of processed foods in the diet.

High-quality, unprocessed carbs, plant-based proteins, and heart-healthy poly- and monounsaturated fats are at the foundation of Blue Zone diets, though macronutrient composition differs. Four are high or very high in carbohydrates, about 65–80% of total calories. Only the Ikarian diet is high in fat due to olive oil (>4 tablespoons daily) along with full-fat dairy, meat, and fish. Moderate-fat diets in Sardinia and Nicoya (~20%) are driven by dairy and meat intakes (and olive oil in Sardinia). In contrast, the Okinawan diet is very low in fat. All have low or moderate protein intake. Other notable elements include generally low calories. Okinawans even have a dietary mantra, *Hara hachi bu*, which roughly translates to, "Stop eating when 80% full." Eating slowly with friends and/or family is also common. Mindful eating practices like these facilitate mild to moderate caloric restriction; this itself is related to longer life and less disease, independent of food composition.

The Blue Zones concept arose from direct observation of and interviews with centenarians across the various regions, stimulating additional hypotheses and epidemiologic research on the role of diet and lifestyle in longevity among the five populations. The Sardinian and Ikarian diets, for instance, include wine in moderation; it's a daily part of the social fabric. Sardinian men spend significant amounts of time walking and hiking the hills while shepherding. Ikarians also participate in daily physical activity, and studies show that they also don't smoke and do socialize frequently, nap regularly, and have low levels of depression.

The Mediterranean diet in general has received extensive research attention. The Seven Countries Study first observed that traditional Greek diets (c.1960) were associated with less chronic disease. While some studies have focused on individual elements like olive oil and wine, others have examined the whole diet. For example, a "Mediterranean diet score" calculated in 1995 quantified eight salient components: ratio of monounsaturated to saturated fat; alcohol; legumes; cereals, bread, and potatoes; fruits; vegetables; meat; and dairy. In this small study across three rural Greek villages, a 1-point increase in the score was associated with a 17% reduction in overall mortality. A striking finding was that significant effects were observed *only* for the whole diet pattern; individual dietary elements showed no association when considered in isolation. Hundreds of observational studies have since confirmed the salutary effects of consuming a Mediterranean diet outside of Greece, including in Australia, Sweden, Denmark, Spain, and the US, among others. RCTs have supported these results and, more recently, identified diet–gene interactions that further scientific understanding of the Mediterranean diet on health and longevity. Other RCTs have corroborated the independent roles of both extra virgin olive oil and wine, due in part due to their high polyphenol content.

Longevity among Seventh-day Adventists has been investigated since the 1970s. Much of the work comes from the Adventist Health Study cohorts, the most recent of which included individuals from churches in the US and Canada. Many studies have compared diet and lifestyle habits among vegetarians and nonvegetarians as some Adventists have omnivorous diets that include meat as well as alcohol. A 2014 analysis of 13 investigations found that vegetarians had a 12% lower risk of mortality compared to nonvegetarians. Individual studies have also revealed protective effects among those consuming varying levels of plant-based diets, whether vegan, vegetarian, pescatarian, or lacto-ovo vegetarian, showing that total abstention from all animal products isn't necessary to gain the benefits of a plant-based diet—though vegans eschewing animal foods had the greatest protection. Additional studies of Adventists in Norway, Brazil, and The Netherlands suggest similar protective effects on mortality compared to non-Adventists, particularly among those who joined the church early, thus establishing a lifetime of healthy (eating) habits.

Okinawans are genetically distinct from other Japanese because of the island's isolation; the ongoing Okinawa Centenarian Study, which began in 1975, has shed light on this population. Genetic components associated with longevity have been identified following the observation that siblings of centenarians also have a high likelihood of reaching age 90. Some biomarker evidence indicates less oxidative stress in centenarians, supporting the free radical theory of aging, perhaps related to the high antioxidant content of the Okinawan diet. Data also suggest that 10–15% CR early in life may be related to longevity, alongside high intakes of foods that mimic the biological anti-aging effects of CR like sweet potatoes, fish, sea vegetables, and turmeric. Mild CR is common in later life as well through the aforementioned practice of *Hara hachi bu*. Surely there are many as-yet-unknown gene–environment interactions that influence longevity among Okinawans, as in other Blue Zones.

Recent studies in Okinawa revealed significant dietary changes during the late 20th century, including more meat and fewer pulses and vegetables. As globalization continued to encroach, Okinawa's diet and lifestyle changed dramatically. Studies of Okinawans today (i.e., babies born post–World War II, many of whom were of low birthweight) now show higher death rates than those living in mainland Japan: today's Okinawa is no longer a Blue Zone.

Few studies have been conducted among Costa Ricans on the Nicoya Peninsula, who descend mainly from Chorotega Indians but also have influences from Spanish colonists and freed African slaves. Costa Ricans, like Sardinians, Ikarians, and Okinawans, were largely cut off from globalization until the mid- to late 20th century. A few studies have identified genetic and molecular biomarkers of longevity, but more research is needed on this unique Latin American population.

Diet provides important insights into longevity but is only part of the picture: the whole lifestyle is greater than the sum of its parts. Physical activity is paramount across the Blue Zones and centers upon walking; activity is generally low intensity, although frequent and built into daily life. (Sardinian shepherds are exceptions.) Movement in general is also common. Okinawans, for instance, usually sit on the floor, forcing mobility throughout the day that promotes agility and flexibility. Stress is managed through such factors as strong family ties—elders are respected members active in raising grandchildren—and a solid network of friends. Church is a focal point among Loma Lindans, while Okinawans have a *moai*, five friends committed to each other for life. Blue Zone centenarians also practice spirituality of some kind, whether through a specific religious organization or belief system or simply by acknowledging ancestors with gratitude. A positive outlook on life also appears vital: even those who have survived wars and food shortages don't dwell on the past and look to the future with hope. These centenarians just seem happy and satisfied with life and make the most with the gifts they've been given despite (often substantial) hardships. Finally, all Blue Zone centenarians articulate a purpose for their life. Each of these elements has its own research base, showing positive associations with overall health, wellbeing, and longevity that, in combination with a plant-based diet, foster longevity.

And, importantly, National Geographic explorer Dan Buettner points out that Blue Zone centenarians laugh often, and much.

What sustainable practices protect people and the planet?

The concept of a "sustainable diet" was developed in 1986, and the nutrition ecology framework was independently developed to incorporate four quadrants: health, environment, economy, and society. The Food and Agriculture Organization of the United Nations (FAO) defines sustainable diets as those with low environmental impacts that also contribute to food and nutrition security and to healthy lives for present and future generations. Specifically, they are "protective and respectful of biodiversity and ecosystems, culturally acceptable, accessible, economically fair and affordable; nutritionally adequate, safe, and healthy; while optimizing natural and human resources."

The most profound changes needed to ensure that contemporary diets are sustainable lie with industry and will most likely be achieved with strong regulations and technologic innovations that address all of the issues discussed herein: reducing greenhouse gas emissions (GHGe); ending reliance on fossil fuels; protecting forests; defending biodiversity; decreasing water, land, and air pollution; managing soil fertility; banning antibiotics and hormones in animals raised in concentrated animal feeding operations (CAFOs) (and eliminating factory farms completely, in time); reducing packaging materials; removing child and slave labor; shielding workers on farms and in factories; and putting an end to food waste. More than one solution is needed to address these complex public health challenges and others across the food system that threaten both people and the planet (see also Chapters 2, 12, and 18).

Still, individual eaters have their own roles to play with each food purchase, each meal, each bite. A 2016 systematic review of

23 studies in countries including the UK, US, Germany, Italy, Spain, Australia, Norway, New Zealand, and others, for instance, shows that vegetarian and vegan diets were most sustainable across a range of measures, and effects decreased as meat intake increased, particularly red meat.[1] While in most cases meat consumption increased per capita land requirements and supported fewer people, modest amounts of meat and dairy were included in sustainable diets in places where land is suitable for grazing cattle but not for growing crops. Ultra-processed foods were also found to be resource-intensive and therefore less sustainable in some studies. Conversely, diets lower in calories were more sustainable, a simple function of reduced consumption.[2] Likewise, a 2012 European Commission (EC) report found that if all Europeans followed low-carbon diets that reduce meat consumption in particular, GHGe would shrink by 30%. Even more striking, the EC and World Wildlife Fund (WWF) found that "[s]imply reducing meat consumption to healthy levels *alone* would achieve nearly all of the emission reductions needed" (emphasis mine). Shifting to plant-based, low-carbon diets often saves money, too, as plant-based proteins are generally less costly than animal proteins—and are also beneficial for health, weight, and longevity.

The clear scientific consensus surrounding the role of diet in climate change in particular has led a host of organizations to incorporate sustainable eating guidelines into their recommendations. FAO, WWF, the World Resources Institute (WRI), the United Nations European Commission, UK's Eating Better alliance (with its 30+ member organizations), the Natural Resources Defense Council, and many individual countries have begun emphasizing eco-conscious food choices in their dietary guidelines. In the UK, for instance, the Eatwell plate was modified to become the LiveWell plate and was subsequently adapted for Sweden, France, and Spain. The US does not highlight the environmental impact of animal consumption in its 2015–2020 dietary guidelines, despite the consensus of its appointed Science Advisory Committee, likely reflecting the influence of the beef and dairy industries on nutrition policy.

The WRI calculated that a significant reduction in beef and animal protein intake among high consumers—which is most Americans, and many Europeans—could spare 310–640 million hectares of land, roughly twice the size of India and more than the entire area of land converted to agricultural use since the 1960s. The associated land use change–related GHGe was a staggering 168 billion tons of carbon dioxide equivalents, more than threefold the total emissions during the entire calendar year of 2009. The report's conclusion is simple yet astonishing: "Reducing consumption of animal-based foods among the world's wealthier populations could free up significant amounts of land—possibly enabling the world to feed 10 billion people by 2050 without agriculture further expanding into forests."[3]

Thus, WRI's three evidence-based guidelines for sustainable eating are: (1) Reduce overconsumption of calories; (2) Reduce overconsumption of protein intake by reducing animal-based foods; and (3) Reduce meat intake, specifically beef. (Note that the first tenet is not encouraging caloric restriction per se but, rather, highlighting that too many people consume excess energy, and each calorie requires substantial energy, land, and water to produce and generates GHGe and other waste byproducts.) There are additional steps eaters can take to reduce their environmental footprint and further FAO's vision of a sustainable diet, too, like drinking tap water when possible (Chapter 14), decreasing food waste (Chapter 2), and limiting foods with excessing packaging (Chapter 4). As important is learning about how your food was produced, including not just the environment but also how your choices impact farmworkers, communities, and other critical concepts discussed throughout this book.

Is dietary change possible?

Taste begins with biology and genetic predisposition (Chapter 5), but dietary preferences are shaped by what mom eats, first transferred by amniotic fluid in utero and later from breast milk. This nature–nurture effect is particularly active in infancy and early childhood and clearly shows that what you eat impacts what you like.[4] Although modifying taste preferences in adulthood is more difficult, and change is never easy, scientific understanding of how taste and food preferences are shaped from both the biological and social sciences demonstrates that diet modification *is* possible.

The key to training your taste buds to prefer healthier foods is, thus, eating them. Try, try again is critical: repeated exposure is essential. Studies suggest that between 6 and 15 distinct experiences are needed, over time, before increased enjoyment and intake are seen. Tasting and smelling the food, not just seeing or learning about it, is necessary at all ages. Associative learning (or conditioning) is also required for older children and adults: an encouraging and supportive social environment, across a variety of settings and dishes, is critical to create a positive taste experience. In time, repeated exposure in positive settings and situations will alter neural pathways in the brain, which can then be reinforced through thoughts and actions. A similar process may be followed to learn to enjoy a less-sweet, less-salty diet: gradually reduce the amount of sugar/salt in in the foods you consume, a little at a time, to give your palate time to adjust.

Unlike children, who are driven mainly by the hedonic effects of food, biology, and early learning, adult diets are also shaped by factors like cost, convenience, and health considerations (Chapter 5); sociocultural influences must also be addressed. And, while nutrition knowledge empowers change for some people, it is seldom adequate to evoke or sustain long-lasting dietary transformation, particularly for most eaters reading this book who live in food-abundant areas with temptations at every turn. Who *doesn't* want another piping hot slice of New York City–style cheese pizza? (I'm talking about myself here.) In other words, modifying your palate is just part of the process; altering environmental cues is critical to make the healthy choice the easy choice through "nudges" that enforce healthy eating.

Taking a step back to consider your current eating pattern is a good place to begin creating a healthier diet. You might begin by asking such questions as: What is your ultimate diet and health goal, and why? What does your current diet look like? What drives your everyday food behavior? Thinking about goals and motivation is also important. Once you've done some dietary detective work and soul-searching, there are mounds of evidence-based strategies to help you in your journey, from creating a more salubrious home food environment to finding social support. Additional strategies, like mindful eating (which brings attentiveness to physical and emotional sensations connected with dining or being in a food environment), are also helpful to some people. (A free infographic is available at pknewby.com.)

But, like all behavior change, you gotta really want it, and patience and perseverance are paramount. Of utmost importance are Winston Churchill's famous words, "Never, never, never give up."

18

THE FUTURE OF FOOD AND NUTRITION

How will we sustainably feed 10 billion people in 2050—and beyond?

Current estimates suggest that about 50% more food, feed, and biofuel is required to nourish about one-third more mouths—almost 10 billion people—in 2050. The Food and Agriculture Organization of the United Nations (FAO) is "cautiously optimistic" that there are sufficient resources globally to meet these needs, though more arable land will be needed in sub-Saharan Africa and Latin America. Some countries in South Asia and the Near East/North Africa have already reached or will soon reach the limits of land available. While water demand will slow due to improvements in irrigation and efficiency, an increase of 11% will still be needed; this will be particularly problematic due to growing water scarcity, which will likely increase as a result of climate change.

FAO predicts that 90% of the additional food will be attained through increased yields, with only 10% from additional land. Other critical elements include increasing access, improving conditions for farmworkers, and investing in agricultural and rural development. Yet additional strategies rely not on increasing supply but, rather, on better utilizing what we have. Cutting global food waste, for example, would significantly decrease the need to produce more food. Indeed, a wide range of organizations have already begun linking sources of food waste with places of food need. FAO also reminds us that if all the crops currently produced for feeding animals—40% of those raised—were instead used directly for human consumption, while available grasslands were used more efficiently for livestock feed, *we would not require additional food to feed 10 billion.*

For these reasons and many others, the scientific consensus is that the world will be fully capable of feeding everyone in the year 2050 (environmental catastrophe notwithstanding), just as it is today. The bigger challenge is whether we can meet those needs sustainably, actualizing FAO's vision of "a world free from hunger and malnutrition, where food and agriculture contribute to improving the living standards of all, especially the poorest, in an economically, socially and environmentally sustainable manner" through its 2030 Agenda for Sustainable Development that envisions "a fairer, more peaceful world in which no one is left behind" (Table 18.1).

There is no single route to sustainability, but there are a variety of agricultural methods underway worldwide. These include, for instance, organic and integrated pest management (IPM; Chapter 2) as well as conservation agriculture, which cultivates diverse farms

Table 18.1 17 Sustainable Development Goals from the Food and Agriculture Organization of the United Nations

1. No poverty
2. Zero hunger
3. Good health and wellbeing
4. Quality education
5. Gender equality
6. Clean water and sanitation
7. Affordable and clean energy
8. Decent work and economic growth
9. Industry, innovation, and infrastructure
10. Reduced inequalities
11. Sustainable cities and communities
12. Responsible consumption and production
13. Climate action
14. Life below water
15. Life on land
16. Peace, justice, and strong institutions
17. Partnerships for the goals

Part of "Transforming Our World: The 2030 Agenda for Sustainable Development" ("2030 Agenda") created by the United Nations in an intergovernmental post-2015 development agenda.

(polyculture) that work with natural ecosystems alongside trees and shrubs (agroforestry) and protects soil using cover crops that contribute to a healthy nitrogen cycle. Agroecology, which FAO defines as "the science of applying ecological concepts and principles to manage interactions between plants, animals, humans and the environment for food security and nutrition," is also on the rise. Agroecology applies traditional and local wisdom to build strong farming systems; it also incorporates food sovereignty and the right to food, human and social values, and cultural and food traditions.

Whatever the system, the changing landscape of farming will give rise to farmers with more specialized knowledge for growing crops. And the increasing use of robotics, like "swarm robots" that carry out tasks collectively, will reduce human labor overall but greatly improve the efficiency and sustainability of tomorrow's farms. At the same time, alternative fuels (e.g., wind, solar, nuclear) will slowly replace carbon-based fossil fuels—and newer ways of generating energy will no doubt be employed moving toward the 22nd century and beyond. The key is creating carbon-neutral farming systems, and there are already a number of small terrestrial and fish farms doing it successfully.

Food processing and packaging will also become greener and smarter. For instance, "active packaging" now maximizes shelf life, quality, and safety through gases, microbials, and other chemicals— think bagged salad—but materials and methods and uses will expand greatly in coming years. "Intelligent packaging" communicates directly to the eater: sensors can detect contamination and prevent foodborne illness, for example. And nanotechnology (molecules <100 nanometers) is currently being used to produce biodegradable packaging that creates less waste and harm to the environment and wildlife, among other applications.

Still, future farming and food system transformations will take us only so far in the quest to feed people healthfully, safely, and sustainably—no different from today's world. Treating food as a basic human right is paramount, as is addressing the underlying socioeconomic issues impacting accessibility and creating nutritional disparities. Reducing conflict and war is essential to prevent treating food as a weapon, a major contributor to human-induced malnutrition and hunger. And without sufficient investment in low- and middle-income countries, FAO estimates that 653 million people *would still be undernourished in 2030 despite an adequate food supply.* Thus, whether 2050, 2100, or beyond, the world will never be fully nourished until poverty is eradicated and peace prevails—no matter how much food is available.

How are high tech and big data changing farming?

Science and technology have assisted farmers throughout history (Chapter 3).[1] Today's farmers obtain information and connect with colleagues using apps and platforms that enable "big data" collection and cross-communication. At the same time, precision agriculture (PA) employs methods like satellite navigation and positioning and sensor technology to produce "more with less" by reducing agricultural (and aquacultural) inputs and hence decreasing environmental insults and waste.

PA is commonly used with vegetable crops, though some model farms are using it in animal husbandry with the help of automatons. Think robots milking cows, which also collect data about the animal's movement, milk production, temperature, health—and about 120 other variables to inform bovine management. (Experts predict that robots will be milking cattle on half of all dairy farms in northwestern Europe by 2025.) PA will also be used increasingly to track crops and animals from farm to fork, improving transparency along the food chain that will enable better detection of and quicker solutions to food safety threats. By 2050, many more "climate-smart" farming technologies will be connected, production through postharvesting, enabling ongoing data collection and sharing via methods utilizing Internet of Things (IoT) and machine learning.

Today's tractors and other farm aids are ever more sophisticated machines that employ robotics to carry out diverse tasks. While many bear some resemblance to their ancestors, "Wall-Ye" looks more akin to a (headless) robot: it's a stout, two-wheeled contraption that traverses vineyards and prunes grapevines, its two extensions resembling very long arms. (Wall-Ye won't pour you a glass of wine, however. Yet.) In another application, Watson is assisting with wine production by getting weather, satellite, and sensor data using NASA satellite imagery from the IBM Cloud to produce wine using 25% less water. As well, agricultural drones, descendants of military aviation technology, now fly 120 meters overhead, using advanced sensors and imaging techniques to monitor crops in ways unavailable to the human eye at ground level and inform PA needs. Another astonishing example of micromanufacturing integrated with complex control systems are "autonomous flying microrobots" (aka, "RoboBee")[2]—which also know how to dive, swim, and explode out of the water before flying again. Potential applications could include crop pollination, a growing need in light of dwindling wild bee and honeybee populations (the latter of which show some signs of slowly rebounding).

Will food production move to cities?

Food production in cities is not a new concept, but rooftop gardens, greenhouses, and the like have become a bigger part of the urban landscape in recent years. The latest example aiming to take urban agriculture to the next level (as it were) is vertical farming, which is similar in philosophy and practice to land-based farming. Unlike plants grown in soil and sunlight, often with fertilizer and pesticides to coax the natural environment into productivity, vertical farms are indoors and employ technologies like aeroponics (roots in air, good for root vegetables), hydroponics (roots in water, good for leafy vegetables and berries), or drip irrigation (roots in vermiculite, where nutrient-filled water is dripped directly onto the stem's base, good for wheat and corn). Seeds are stacked vertically in beds, residing in a meticulously controlled climate that enables growth without soil or pesticides. Artificial lights, often LEDs, provide the radiation needed for photosynthesis. One American company also employs "schleppers," tiny robots that navigate the dense network of plants that humans are unable to reach. Altogether, vertical farms use far less water than agriculture and don't produce runoff that erodes soil and damages waterways and ecosystems. They're also safer environments for farmworkers and provide employment in cities, where populations are skyrocketing.

The first vertical farm in the US popped up in 2011, using technology that emerged from growing food on the moon in similar enclosed spaces; the whole system utilizes big data, IoT technology, apps, and other methods to tightly control the environment at all times. Still, vertical farming does not yet lend itself to producing an array of foods that adequately addresses food insecurity and nutritional needs. Nor is it yet suitable for tall crops like cereal grains, which are dietary staples around the world. It is also energy-intensive due to its reliance on artificial light and energy-gobbling systems needed to maintain the indoor growing environment. Vertical farms are costly to develop and manage, too, and don't help destitute rural farmers or revitalize land-based agriculture (though that is obviously not their intent). Another major issue is that vertical farming technicians who praise the "local" aspect of the produce as being more climate-friendly ignore the most dominant factor responsible for energy use and greenhouse gas emissions, which is production, not transportation. Still, it is easy to imagine a future filled with skyscraper-like vertical farms growing diverse crops and powered by wind and energy that reuse biomass in an aquaculture system—and also includes facilities for shipping, shopping, and eating. Perhaps such farms will one day supplant gargantuan feed lots (horizontal farming?) once they're eliminated from tomorrow's food systems.

Will genetic engineering of food continue?

Doubtless there will always be opponents to genetic engineering (GE). Indeed, there are still those who oppose pasteurization, a century hence (!). While vigilance in research, development, regulation, and application is needed for each new seed, the coming decades will see an increasing proportion of crops grown using GE and other advanced, unknown biotech methods—whether to improve nutritional value, deliver medicines or vaccines, combat environmental challenges, or address some other need or desire.

There are, for example, farmers in Uganda who have been yearning to use GE seeds to fight banana bacterial wilt, which wiped out many farms in a situation analogous to the deadly ring spot virus that struck the papaya industry in Hawaii in the late 1990s. Yet biotech was prohibited in Uganda, as it is in many other countries in Africa, largely due to misinformation and myths surrounding the technology (and the politics therein). While treating banana wilt is possible with conventional methods, the cost is prohibitive for Uganda's impoverished farmers. Uganda finally approved the use of GE in

December 2017, paving the road for a "golden banana" that is resistant to wilt—and contains vitamin A, a nutrient in which 30% of Ugandans are deficient. Perhaps the yellow(er) fruit, destined for distribution in 2021, will support destitute farmers, provide a life-saving vitamin to eaters, and facilitate acceptance in other parts of Africa. As more and more positive examples of biotech mount, resistance to the technology will eventually subside and science will prevail, just as it did in Hawaii: the rainbow papaya literally saved the industry and the farmers growing the fruit and is still on supermarket shelves today.

Thus, while the battles have raged concerning genetically modified organisms (GMOs) for the better part of three decades—and remain heated even in Hawaii, despite the GE papaya's success—the tide will slowly change as the century progresses. By 2050, GE methods will be a regular part of the go-to toolkit for sustainable farming around the world. After all, GE seeds are still seeds: they too can be grown using sustainable methods that embrace agroecology ideals. "GMOrganic" or "AgroGMO" will certainly be a part of the future of food—and it's already in use in some places.

Will animals still be raised for food?

Gene Roddenberry was hardly the first to raise the ethics of eating animals in light of viable alternatives in *Star Trek's* sci-fi, 24th-century universe.[3] In 1930, Winston Churchill opined, "Fifty years hence, we shall escape the absurdity of growing a whole chicken in order to eat the breast or wing by growing these parts separately under a suitable medium." Chemist Pierre Eugène Marcellin Berthelot also claimed, in 1894, that humans would consume meat produced in a lab rather than from animals by the year 2000 based on his then radical belief that anything organic (carbon-based) could be synthesized. And many throughout history have championed the power of plants over animals, including Albert Einstein, who famously stated, "Nothing will benefit health or increase chances of survival on earth as the evolution to a vegetarian diet."

As the decades progress, animals will remain part of the human diet to some degree, particularly where they are part of ecologically sound systems critical to local livelihoods and survival. Insects will also continue to play some a role. Even so, the human taste for animal flesh and products will gradually decrease in centuries' time, as meat alternatives become tastier and better accepted. This may result from awakening environmental consciousness and changing philosophical proclivities surrounding food choices that lead to lower demand—consider the growth of the non-dairy milk market in the US, for example—or decreased supply due to catastrophic events.

Two of today's technologies aim to create meat alternatives by sidestepping the farm altogether. In the first method, plant proteins are used to create meat-like foods to provide non–meat eaters with more protein choices (think about the now decades-old familiar veggie burger). The newest additions to the market begin with plant proteins, often pea, and use a better recipe that creates a meatier texture and mouth feel. Beetroot juice is used in some products, yielding a moist, pink interior that "bleeds" when cooked. Others use a plant-based version of heme iron, the same compound found in animals that gives meat its red color and umami taste.

The second method creates animal foods in the lab. Like many technologies, the idea of growing meat without animals began in NASA more than two decades ago as a way to feed astronauts en route to Mars. Names are many: clean meat, lab meat, cultured meat, in vitro meat (IVM), finless fish. The process, cellular agriculture, employs the same underlying philosophy as traditional agriculture—creating higher yields with fewer resources—sans animals. The first food, a hamburger, was made in The Netherlands in 2013, proof of concept that meat could be grown outside of an animal and without pain or slaughter.[4] The same IVM methods are being used to produce chicken, duck, liver, and fish—as well as dairy products like yogurt and eggs. Still, it will take some time for IVM to disrupt the beef market significantly. Efforts are thus far confined to individual laboratories solving the science, with particular attention to developing nonanimal media. Large-scale production of cultured meat of any kind will also require enormous bioreactors to culture the cells—think large stainless steel vats for brewing beer. This process will also require energy, although it will carry much lower environmental and other costs compared to raising and eating animals.

Will animal farming become victim to the same fate as so many other industries that, over time, either fail to meet a need, are replaced with better options, or are simply so detrimental to health and society that they eventually die? (The coal industry comes to mind, as does the horse and buggy.) It may be quite some time before IVM and other alternatives supplant the real thing: the taste for meat is strong in Western diets and is escalating around the world, particularly in China. Nevertheless, surveys found that about 75% of consumers in Belgium and The Netherlands and 65% in the US were willing to try IVM. The trend will continue to grow with the next generation of eaters who will be less frightened of technology and more willing to try new foods. And with places like China investing heavily in cultured meat, we just may be able to reshape the palate of tomorrow's eater.

Is "personalized nutrition" hope or hype?

Despite the similarity in nutrient needs across species—*Homo sapiens* are, in fact, 99.9% alike—we nonetheless have genetic variability. The exhilarating progression of genetic research in general, and diet–gene studies specifically, has spurred great interest in personalized nutrition (aka, precision nutrition), which promises individualized dietary advice tailored to your genome.[5] Some studies support a personalized nutrition approach to obesity, for example, as there are a number of genes whose variants play a role in diet and nutrient metabolism, hence weight.

In 2006, the US Government Accountability Office submitted a report calling out four companies for misleading consumers about what personalized programs can really offer. Yet, by 2017, more than a dozen companies marketed such programs, though there remain several chief issues compromising their effectiveness. A major challenge is that most chronic, noncommunicable diseases involve many genes interacting with each other as well as a host of environmental influences—of which diet is just one. Reductionist thinking often misses critical elements in complex systems, either because they are unaccounted for or as yet unknown. A 2015 meta-analysis on 524 592 individuals and 38 genes found no significant associations with either diet intakes or a range of nutritional disorders, suggesting that consumers employing individual nutrigenomic testing to provide a personalized nutrition plan may not lead to desired effects at this stage of the science. The ongoing Food4Me randomized controlled trial (RCT) of European adults has provided important insights about whether giving genotype and phenotype (biomarkers, weight, etc.) information to eaters alters dietary intakes, weight, and blood pressure. After many studies, the authors concluded that knowing one's genes does not meaningfully impact behavior change. Indeed, their findings are consistent with decades of health behavior research showing again and again that information alone is rarely sufficient to create behavior change—particularly without other interventions.

Therefore, despite the titillating notion of obtaining a diet regimen designed perfectly for you, your personal genome is just one piece of the puzzle. And, perhaps most critically, even perfectly precise nutrition, once it exists—which will be quite some time—won't eliminate the need for behavior change. Diet advice will always compete with other factors. Thus, even when a personalized nutrition program is available for every person (who can afford it), considerable effort will remain to implement the plan in a way that works alongside other lifestyle factors that shape everyday eating behavior.

What will dinner look like?

Homo sapiens will evolve toward a diet filled with a greater quantity and variety of plants of all kinds; seaweed and microalgae (e.g., spirulina), collectively often referred to as "algae" (Chapter 9), will play a major role. Microalgae are easy to grow and can be used as food for humans, biomass for animal feed, or a source of biofuel. Some species are also able to fix carbon dioxide, a potential boon to combating climate change. Algae also absorb heavy metals and remove excess nitrogen and phosphate to help clean wastewater; algal ponds for such uses already exist and will continue to grow in number and magnitude. Although a number of factors are currently limiting algae's potential, including extraction and purification costs and large-scale application for its various products and byproducts across industries, the market will soon explode through algal biofactories that contribute to sustainability in myriad ways.

We will also continue finding new foods in nature. In fact, most scientists agree that the vast majority of life on Earth is undiscovered, including edible flora. It's a big world with much to nosh that we've never even tried. Diets in high-income nations slowly evolve over time when new foods are explored in different cultures and eventually gain global popularity. Many so-called "ethnic" foods—pizza, salsa, Chinese food—were brought to the US, for example, and are now favorites here, and elsewhere. In tomorrow's supper, perhaps the same will be said of insects, which are already consumed by about 2 billion people worldwide by choice, not necessity, providing valuable protein and a range of nutrients at a fraction of the environmental cost of raising mammals and other animals.

Other major changes in human diets will emerge not from nature, but from technology. It is hard to imagine what such foods may look like. Could anyone have predicted a Twinkie? Or a vitamin-fortified sports bar? Yet what is certain is that changing lifestyles, increasing knowledge, and advancing technology will give rise to ever more novel foodstuffs, just as it has throughout history.

How will machines change how we cook and eat?

Like farming, cooking will certainly continue to some degree: it does so even in *Star Trek*'s 24th century, although most victuals come from a no-prep-required food replicator. Still then do arguments remain over the role the machine should play in food production—certainly fresh-from-the-farm, home-cooked meals are superior!—to illuminate the juxtaposing viewpoints that have always been, and will always be, part of social discourse whenever new technologies arise.

Robotics in particular will alter the way we eat. The early 21st century saw restaurants without any human involvement arise—at least, on the front end. The first was Robot Kitchen in Hong Kong in 2006, featuring two robots (cleverly named Robot 1 and Robot 2) that recognize voice patterns, take meal orders, send them by infrared to human kitchen cooks, and deliver them to the table using a video camera that detects objects in its path. A third robot was later designed to flip burgers and make omelets. Since then, more and more restaurants have sprung up in China and Japan, with a few in the US and Europe. And it's only a matter of time before robots are making home meals—at least, for those who can afford them. Moley Robotics will soon launch "the world's first fully-automated and integrated intelligent cooking robot." (The price tag is $92K.) The user begins by specifying the number of desired portions, cuisine preference, preferred ingredients, calories, dietary restrictions, cooking method, and specific chef. Humans need only procure the ingredients and slot them in, and away it cooks.

It will be quite some time before robots are readily available to and affordable for everyday eaters. Until then, 3D food printers (Chapter 3), "smart ovens," or digital scales may enter your kitchen, interconnected with your computer, through Internet of Things (IoT, aka "machine learning") technology. IoT will monitor the pantry and fridge, signal the need to restock, and place the order for delivery, which will also be useful in institutional and restaurant settings. Or perhaps you could order takeout—and a robot will bring it to your door. (This, too, already exists.) In time, IoT will create a food profile of your preferences and habits to help direct your eating habits; it will be far more comprehensive than current apps and integrated fully with your personal health profile.

Indeed, the number of machines popping up to handle shopping, prep, cooking, and cleanup using IoT technology is staggering. Interestingly, among the top sellers are those informing you when foods are "expired". Yet given that expiration dates are not an indicator of food safety, or even food quality, such a device actually encourages food waste. Hence the "GIGO" (garbage in, garbage out) principle pertains here as everywhere: "smart" anything is dependent on the accuracy of the data. There are already a great many junk science products leading consumers astray, particularly when it comes to food and nutrition; the Internet of (food and nutrition) Things will magnify that problem if machines are not evidence-based.

What does food evolution look like?

Nutrition science will continue to evolve, discovering even more reasons why what we eat matters, from farm to fork, and revealing ever more ways to promote health, prevent disease, and live longer. And through advancing science-based dietary guidelines and evidence-based recommendations, individuals will be even more knowledgeable about how to make the best choices for their bodies and our planet. Food environments will become healthier in time, too, with more nutrient-dense, plant-based options offered across the board, from schools to restaurants, hospitals to workplaces. Thus, for those well informed and with sufficient incentive and wherewithal (not to mention adequate fiscal resources), creating a salubrious diet comprising the most nutritious and sustainable food choices will always be an option.

Just as it is today.

Yet IoT technology will continue to make healthy and sustainable eating easier to enact throughout the 21st century by connecting the quantified self with quantified food. In other words, emerging and novel technologies will connect big data about your diet and life-style with your overall health and wellbeing, whatever your interest (e.g., weight loss, work productivity, athletic performance, sleep quality, improved mood, living longer, preventing disease)—and it will all be quantified, available, and interconnected across myriad machines. You'll be able to measure all of the details about your diet with ease, for example—and tomorrow's technologies will be smart enough to measure what you're eating directly, likely from internal sensors, with no need to enter subjectively recalled food data manually, as with current apps. Nutritional information could then be shared with your kitchen appliances or might pop up in your smart phone to facilitate wiser choices, wherever you are. These data will also be part of your comprehensive health profile, where you can measure and monitor impacts over time, if you wish. This is just the beginning: your machines may also be part of a smart home, or a smart community, in which big data will facilitate even more opportunities to live your healthiest life.

Yet however sophisticated IoT becomes, no matter how much data are provided across how many platforms, food temptations will always exist to compete with our interest in health. (At least, I hope so.) And there is little reason to believe that future humans will be any more interested in changing nutrition behavior than those in the present. Therefore, improvements to health and disease will come not from behavior change but from large-scale changes to food production through modifications to business-as-usual models in which food systems create better choices, consumer unawares.

Other significant changes to diet-related health will emerge due to nutrification (Chapter 6), which will long continue: it is simply the best way to change the health trajectory of a population. One early 21st century product, Soylent, is a meal-replacement shake that provides complete nutritional value. It's also relatively inexpensive and vegan and uses compostable containers; thus, it's both consumer- and environmentally friendly. It's a favorite among those who have no interest in cooking meals or contemplating nutrition but still want to be healthy. And it was so popular online that it came to brick-and-mortar stores after only several years. Still, its reductionist approach misses the mark on the state of the science. Namely, the whole diet is greater than the sum of its parts: a plant-based, nutrient-rich diet filled with a variety of minimally processed foods provides an array of elements known, *and unknown*, that foster health, disease prevention, and longevity. Still, Soylent (and other products like it) is a more nutritious and sustainable choice compared to most Western diets, limitations notwithstanding.

While current "one size fits all" approaches like Soylent are intriguing examples of nutrification, most people just don't want that kind of meal. Moreover, the (distant) future is precision nutrition. Will it be an elixir in and of itself? No, because complex diseases arise from many more elements than just diet. But will personalized nutrition plans enable better protection from chronic diseases like heart disease, stroke, cancer, Alzheimer's, hypertension, depression, Parkinson's, arthritis, and obesity? And slow down aging? And work with your brain's specific chemistry to enhance mental health and mood (and, perhaps, sex drive)? Absolutely. In time, science will offer very specific dietary answers to manage individual susceptibility—for those inclined to follow one. And, for others, broad-scale fortification programs will quietly continue to nutrify the food supply, facilitating better health without requiring behavior change. Additional interventions remain unknown, but some variant of *Star Trek*'s food replicator, dispensing perfectly and personally nutrified food—*and* chocolate ice cream—seems certain.

Because if nutrition isn't used to help make people healthier, and the ultimate goal isn't to eradicate disease and enable optimal health and wellbeing and a long life in all the ways we can, with all the means we can, what's the point?

NOTES

CHAPTER 2

1 "Famine" is defined by the Food and Agriculture Organization of the United Nations [FAO] as widespread food shortages that cause more than 30% of children under age 5 to suffer from acute malnutrition, with mortality rates of 2 or more people per 10 000 daily, among other criteria.

2 NASA estimates that humans have increased atmospheric CO_2 by more than a third since the beginning of the Industrial Revolution, calling it "the most important long-lived 'forcing' of climate change" due chiefly to burning oil, coal, and natural gas, which combines with atmospheric oxygen to form CO_2. The US Department of Energy estimated that China was responsible for the largest contribution to global CO_2 emissions in 2017 (30%), while the US was second (15%) and the EU third (9%); India (7%), the Russian Federation (5%), and Japan (4%) follow. All other countries where data are available contribute 30% of emissions, in aggregate.

3 A study comparing zinc bioavailability to requirements across various crops in 188 countries quantified those at risk of deficiency under normal and elevated CO_2 concentrations at levels expected in 2050: an additional 138 million were found to be at risk under these conditions, mostly in Africa, South Asia, and India.

4 Ropelk again writes, "The decimation of giant bluefin is emblematic of everything wrong with global fisheries today: the vastly increased killing power of new fishing technology, the shadowy network of international companies making huge profits from the trade, negligent fisheries management and enforcement, and consumers' indifference to the fate of the fish they choose to buy."

CHAPTER 3

1 A recent anthropological study revealed that eating fruit in particular was associated with larger brain size in 140 nonhuman primate species compared to meat or leaves, suggesting that diet rather than social organization (the "social brain" hypothesis) was the critical factor fueling

brain growth. Whether the effect was due to fruit's rich set of nutrients and phytochemicals or the difficulty in fruit foraging is unclear; both were likely important. As Bret Stitka writes, "Being able to find, pick, and peel a dangling passion fruit takes a lot more brainpower than simply tearing off leaves."

2 The ability to use both tools and heat in food preparation and consumption together during the Paleolithic period became increasingly common as evolution progressed, leading to such anthropometric changes as stronger bones, smaller teeth, and larger skulls, to house 300% (!) bigger brains. Various factors have been hypothesized to boost brain growth beyond cooking, including omega-3 fatty acids found in seafood (Chapter 8). Doubtless, the process of developing tools itself was also critical: creating gizmos may have been either a cause or an effect of larger brain size (or both).

3 There are numerous other examples of preagricultural sedentism by foragers, many of whom also engaged in crafts, including another hunter–gatherer settlement located in modern Turkey going back 11 000 years. In other words, agriculture did not always predate settlements, nor were the two always hand in hand: neither agriculture nor city-states were required for rich civilizations to develop. Other studies suggest that the presence of animals in early farming activities was the cornerstone of social inequalities, particularly in Old World Neolithic settlements: those who owned animals were able to farm ever larger swaths of land, growing and storing more food and accumulating greater wealth. Land and animals were then passed on through generations, creating larger socioeconomic divisions between workers and owners. Finally, grain was fundamental to the later development of city-states: it was used as a form of currency and was also easily taxed (later codified and quantified through writing).

4 Canning came about when the French government offered money for a method to get foods safely to Napoleon's troops during the war. Inventor Nicholas Appert discovered that heating foods in airtight containers kept them safe to eat, winning the cash prize in 1795. Though Appert originally used glass jars, the process was later reproduced with metal in England in 1810, making its way to the US in 1821.

5 Swill milk was common for several decades in 19th-century New York City, a result of milk produced from cows living near city distilleries that were fed leftover alcoholic mash from whiskey-making. The bluish liquid was then mixed with plaster of Paris, starch, eggs, and molasses to give it the "buttercup hue" like that arriving from Westchester and Orange Counties, the common origin of milk at the time. The *New York Times* reported that up to 8000 children died as a result of drinking swill milk.

6 Dr. Norman Borlaug was a plant pathologist and geneticist who developed "semi-dwarf" wheat varieties (1944) that were more disease-resistant and therefore showed significantly higher yields than their traditional counterparts. As a result, wheat production more than doubled where these techniques were introduced, mainly the US, Mexico, and Latin America; rice production also increased considerably in India, South Asia, and Southeast Asia. Borlaug received the Nobel Peace Prize in 1970 for his role

in increasing food security and preventing starvation, credited today by many as "the man who saved a billion lives." Yet gains were not realized globally, and efforts to get these agricultural advances to Africa didn't begin in earnest until the new millennium.

7 The primary use of DDT (dichlorodiphenyltrichloroethane) was in preventing malaria, typhus, and other insect-borne diseases, for which it was extremely effective. As its use proliferated in farming and animal husbandry, as well as in home gardens, adverse effects on wildlife and human health mounted. DDT was later determined to be a "probable carcinogen" and was banned by EPA in 1972; it is no longer permitted in the agricultural sector in any setting. DDT is still approved by WHO and others for use in indoor environments to control malaria, however, with the belief that the human health benefits in preventing this disease endemic in many parts of Africa outweigh the potential environmental harms when used properly.

CHAPTER 4

1 Heme iron is found in animal protein foods and accounts for 95% of the iron in the human body. It is more easily absorbed by the body (bioavailable) than non-heme, the kind found dominantly in plant foods. Heme may interact with other diet components in the body to raise cancer risk, perhaps synergistically. One study suggests that effects may be enhanced with higher-fat meats, for example.

2 Ongoing vigilance is nonetheless critical, as with any new and still evolving technology. One particular concern is that GE arises from a reductionist philosophy, which can unwittingly lead to negative externalities in light of incomplete knowledge. Minute changes—genetic edits—may cause unintended effects that disrupt the larger (eco)system or whole organism. Though current evidence for the safety of GE plants and salmon is solid, risks may increase as biotech methods are applied in more complex settings and species.

3 A 2016 study of more than 3000 Scottish Atlantic salmon farmed between 2006 and 2015 reported that EPA and DHA concentrations decreased by more than half on average from 2010 on, when fish oil used in feed decreased—though the omega-3 content was still higher than in Norwegian farmed salmon. This is because many Scottish salmon farms still use some fish oil in the feed, while Norwegian salmon operations have increased their reliance on more sustainable plant-based feeds. EPA and DHA content of Australian farmed salmon similarly decreased due to the switch in feed from fish oil to poultry oil—but was still higher than that in wild salmon.

4 The authors hypothesize, "In most mammals, including rats and humans, sweet receptors evolved in ancestral environments poor in sugars and are thus not adapted to high concentrations of sweet tastants. The supranormal stimulation of these receptors by sugar-rich diets, such as those now widely available in modern societies, would generate a supranormal reward signal in the brain, with the potential to override self-control mechanisms and thus lead to addiction."

5   Breast milk also includes 0.9–1.2 g/dL protein (mostly casein, α-lactalbumin, lactoferrin, secretory immunoglobulin A, lysozyme, and serum albumin, plus non-protein nitrogen-containing compounds like urea, uric acid, creatine, creatinine, amino acids, and nucleotides); 3.2–3.6 g/dL fat (palmitic and oleic acids); and 6.7–7.8 g/dL carbohydrate. As children age, breast milk is a significant source of calories and nutrients, around half until 12 months—as "complementary feeding" of solid foods begins at around 6 months, when nutritional needs exceed what breast milk alone can provide—and one-third at 12–24 months.

6   Wet nurses were the logical (and usual) alternative, when available. Archaeological evidence of prehistoric baby bottles suggestive of "artificial feeding" dates back to the Bronze Age. Cow's milk (2nd century BCE), other animal milk, prechewed food, and mixtures of grains with water or broth were common, as were other concoctions. These alternatives did not provide comparable nutrition—or immunologic protection—of breast milk, and those children had poorer survival. During the Industrial Revolution, infections ran rampant in urban slums, yet fewer children were breastfed since women earned more money working in factories than as wet nurses.

CHAPTER 5

1   The variability of food preferences across the globe has stimulated a large body of literature examining whether taste is learned or innate. One small study compared eaters and non-eaters of spicy foods across a range of sensory, physiological, personality, and cultural factors. It showed no sensory and physiological differences in perception. Rather, aficionados had been consuming spicy food since childhood, reflecting learned behavior. Another study examined how people ranked the burn and bitterness across eight samples of capsaicin (the chemical responsible for the warming effect of spicy foods) that differed in heat intensity. Variables like intake frequency, experience, and personality factors were studied to evaluate whether the "chronic desensitization hypothesis" was a driving explanation for spicy food consumption. Results showed that personality factors like sensation seeking and sensitivity to reward were major drivers and that, while eating spicy foods was correlated with learned behavior, eaters did not objectively experience the heat any differently from non-eaters. Some just like it hot, it seems.

2   Advertising has evolved, but the concept isn't new—and neither are efforts to curtail its impact on children. In 1874, the British Parliament passed legislation to protect England's youngest citizens from street merchants hocking kid-friendly products. Advertising methods have grown greatly in the century and a half since, taking the form of television commercials, product placements, Google ads, highway billboards, celebrity endorsements, and the like.

3   The National School Lunch Act was passed in 1946 "to safeguard the health and wellbeing of the Nation's children and to encourage the domestic consumption of nutritious agricultural commodities and other food." During its first year, the National School Lunch Program (NSLP) operated in 44 537 schools and served 910.9 million meals to 6 million children, rising

to 79 000 schools, 24.5 million children, and 3 billion meals in 1971. Other programs were later developed to meet nutritional needs in schools and similar organizations, particularly among low-income individuals, including the School Breakfast Program, the Child and Adult Care Food Program, the Summer Food Service Program, and the Special Milk Program; each is administered through the states, which are reimbursed if they follow federal guidelines (e.g., nutritional standards).

4 Remember the old American-style Westerns with chuckwagons? These food truck progenitors and their "cookies" (cooks) provided essential nourishment to those heading west during the Gold Rush (1848–1855) or fighting the Civil War (1861–1865). City folk had their own variant in the form of the pushcart, an early ancestor of today's corner food carts (think hot dogs in New York City) sans cooking functionality that fed workers during the Industrial Revolution. The iconic ice cream truck with its Good Humor "ice cream on a stick" pops was born in 1920 and is still around today, followed by larger taco- and burger-selling outfits, once known as "roach coaches" for their less-than-stellar food hygiene practices.

CHAPTER 8

1 EFSA concluded that glycidol, a byproduct of palm oil when processed above 200°C, is carcinogenic and genotoxic. Similar byproducts can be found in other vegetable fats, though palm oil yields the most. However, many industries specifically do not process palm oil at these temperatures for that reason; thus, other organizations, like both WHO and FDA, have not raised similar concerns about glycidol and palm oil.

2 Other potential names under which palm oil may be hidden include vegetable fat, palm kernel, palm kernel oil, palm fruit oil, palmate, palmitate, palmolein, glyceryl, stearate, stearic acid, *Elaeis guineensis*, palmitic acid, palm stearine, palmitoyl oxostearamide, palmitoyl tetrapeptide-3, sodium laureth sulfate, sodium lauryl sulfate, sodium kernelate, sodium palm kernelate, sodium lauryl lactylate/sulfate, hydrated palm glycerides, ethyl palmitate, and octyl palmitate. Whew!

CHAPTER 9

1 Apples do contain pesticide residues, like most produce; and some are contaminated with heavy metals. Comprehensive risk scenarios were investigated across 696 samples for 182 pesticides in Poland, and researchers found that chronic and acute exposures due to apple consumption were within acceptable limits based on current safety regulations and should not pose a health risk to either children or adults. Apples in China also revealed heavy-metal contamination using soil pollution and health risk indices, though metals were found to be in an acceptable range with no excess health risk. Despite the media attention that studies like these often evoke, the health benefits of eating apples likely far outweigh any potential risk from pesticide or heavy-metal contamination.

2 The German Nutrition Study is particularly noteworthy due to the strength of its methods and study design. RCTs and meta-studies were given greater

weight compared to individual observational studies, for example. As well, a much broader array of studies was included compared to the other analyses.

CHAPTER 10

1 Null study results do not always reflect a true lack of association in scientific studies. For example, a recent RCT of whole grains observed dietary noncompliance, in which participants were not consuming the amount of whole grains they were told to eat. Noncompliance biases findings since the groups no longer look different. This is why nutrition scientists are always seeking more precise biological measures that objectively measure dietary intakes, which are known as "biomarkers." Biomarkers do not exist for many dietary components, however, and are thus an active research area since they strengthen the veracity of a study's findings when used.

CHAPTER 12

1 The growing scarcity of water has stimulated more research focused on the water footprint of various animal and plant products. Three components contribute to a crop's water footprint: green water (rainwater), blue water (surface and groundwater), and gray water (due to pollution of surface or groundwater). The extensive use of blue water in agriculture is particularly concerning given that the rate of withdrawal from aquifers currently exceeds replenishment.

2 A 2015 report concluded that the bacterium *Lactobacillus rhamnosus* GG (LGG), isolated about two decades ago, is a prototypical strain given its clinical impact, including its high adhesion rate, resistance against gastric acidity, and antimicrobial activity against pathogens (e.g., *Salmonella*). LGG has been effective for eradication of *Helicobacter pylori*, for example, which causes stomach ulcers.

3 Ameraucana chickens (an American breed that hails from its Chilean cousin, Araucana) produce lovely blue eggs. While some of the chickens do indeed come in shades of blue, however, they may also be silver, white, or some other color; it's the breed's gene that leads to the blue eggs, not (necessarily) the color of its feathers.

CHAPTER 14

1 Much of this excellent information comes from a 2016 article in the *New York Times*, which allows readers to quantify their environmental impact from bottled water consumption. Check it out, and share with your friends: https://www.nytimes.com/interactive/2016/science/bottled-water-or-tap.html.

CHAPTER 17

1 Additional studies further considered the practicality of sustainable diets for consumers when compared to general consumption habits and cost. One such examined whether diets with commonly consumed foods in the

UK could lower GHGe. Results showed that a realistic diet that included 52 foods and less meat but was otherwise similar to common British diet patterns showed a 36% reduction in GHGe at similar food cost. Similarly, a study examining common diets in French adults indicated that the most sustainable diets were higher in plant foods and overall nutrition quality yet lower in total calories, energy density, cost, and GHGe. In yet another study, simulations where average Americans cut meat/dairy/fish/egg consumption in half reduced per person land use and agricultural GHGe by almost 50%.

2 The majority of nutrition studies on sustainable eating are focused on Western diets, including the Mediterranean diet, reflecting the Eurocentric bias of scientific research. No studies have considered the sustainability of the Nicoyan diet, and only one has considered the Japanese diet, reporting a lower nitrogen footprint of traditional diets compared to diets today. Yet, *absence of evidence is not evidence of absence* (a scientific maxim worth remembering): there is no reason to think that other Blue Zone diets low in meat and calories—and other diets with similar composition—should not be similarly sustainable.

3 Addressing diets in the developing world is nonetheless critical given increasing meat and dairy intake: animal food consumption is predicted to increase 80% and beef specifically to rise 95% by 2050, driven mainly by low- and middle-income nations. The move from traditional to Western diets will further compromise sustainability due to such factors as increased refrigeration, which carries with it an energy cost, and loss of biodiversity, which compromises both dietary variety and natural habitats. Water use is of particular concern. In India, for example, agriculture accounts for 90% of freshwater use, and its supplies are increasingly being challenged, as elsewhere. Growing urbanization and other changes will further stress water supplies and will also increase GHGe.

4 Verbal affirmations and parents modeling enjoyment of healthy foods are also important for children.

CHAPTER 18

1 Crop yields in the developing world are generally less than those in the developed world. For example, 1.54 tons of wheat per hectare were produced in low-income countries, 2.74 in middle-income countries, and 8.99 in high-income countries between 2001 and 2012. Gaps between actual and potential yields for some crops are as high as 76% in sub-Saharan Africa and reflect not only insufficient adoption of more productive technologies, according to FAO, but also a lack of market integration and persistent gender inequality that pervade small-scale family farming. Upgrades to cleaner and smarter methods that increase efficiency while also preserving scarce natural resources and reducing food loss and waste are urgently needed in low- and middle-income countries, which are particularly prone to extreme weather events.

2 The project integrated three main components: brain, body, and colony. "Body development consists of constructing robotic insects able to fly on their own with the help of a compact and seamlessly integrated power

source; brain development is concerned with 'smart' sensors and control electronics that mimic the eyes and antennae of a bee, and can sense and respond dynamically to the environment; the Colony's focus is about coordinating the behavior of many independent robots so they act as an effective unit."

3 Science fiction enthusiasts may recall an episode of *Star Trek: The Next Generation* (1987–1994), in which Commander William T. Riker informed an alien visitor that the meat on the starship *U.S.S. Enterprise* did not come from slaughtering animals. Rather, it was obtained through a food replicator, which dematerialized matter and reconstituted it into fare that fed hungry space explorers.

4 The burger comprised about 20 000 strands of muscle grown in cell cultures. The method was not new and has been used in medicine for some years, but this was the first ever application to food (that went prime time, in any case). A medium is nonetheless necessary to initiate cell division. Some producers use fetal bovine serum, an inexpensive byproduct of the livestock industry that ultimately fails to address the bigger issue of using animals for food. Others use stem cells painlessly biopsied from an adult cow. Tissue engineer and physician Mark Post initially used cells removed from dead cows in a slaughterhouse, though he's currently developing the technology to grow muscle strands in bovine-free media.

5 Differences can occur due to either genetic variation in dietary responses (nutrigenetics) or how nutrients and phytochemicals affect gene expression (nutrigenomics). Various other "omics" fields have sprung up to denote where along the genetic path effects occur, whether at the level of ribonucleic acid (RNA) expression (transcriptomics), protein expression (proteomics), or metabolites (metabolomics). The impact of diet on genes at any of these levels can be studied either separately or together to further elucidate heath and disease processes and could theoretically be used to alter one's genetic susceptibility with the "right" diet—ergo, personalized nutrition (aka, precision nutrition).

SELECTED REFERENCES

CHAPTER 1

Coalition of Immokalee Workers. About CIW. http://www.ciw-online.org/about/. Accessed December 5, 2017.

Food and Agriculture Organization of the United Nations. The state of food and agriculture. http://www.fao.org/publications/sofa/2014/en/. Published 2014. Accessed February 10, 2018.

International Labour Organization. Forced labour, modern slavery, and human trafficking. http://www.ilo.org/global/topics/forced-labour/lang--en/index.htm/. Published 2017. Accessed December 5, 2017.

CHAPTER 2

Food and Agriculture Organization of the United Nations. Livestock's long shadow. http://www.fao.org/docrep/010/a0701e/a0701e.pdf. Published 2006. Accessed December 11, 2017.

Food and Agriculture Organization of the United Nations. The state of world fisheries and agriculture: contributing to food security and nutrition for all. http://www.fao.org/3/a-i5555e.pdf. Published 2016. Accessed September 25, 2017.

Gunders D. Wasted: how America is losing up to 40 percent of its food from farm to fork to landfill. NRDC Issue Paper. Natural Resources Defense Council. https://www.nrdc.org/sites/default/files/wasted-food-IP.pdf. Published August 2012. Accessed October 12, 2017.

Natural Resources Defense Council and Harvard Food Law and Policy Clinic. The dating game: how confusing food date labels lead to food waste in America. http://www.chlpi.org/wp-content/uploads/2013/12/dating-game-report.pdf. Published September 2013. Accessed October 12, 2017.

US Environmental Protection Agency. Global greenhouse gas emissions data. http://www3.epa.gov/climatechange/ghgemissions/global.html. Updated April 13, 2017. Accessed September 27, 2017.

CHAPTER 3

Collyer B. The real roots of early city states may rip up the textbooks. *New Scientist.* October 4, 2017. https://www.newscientist.com/article/mg23631462-700-the-real-roots-of-early-city-states-may-rip-up-the-textbooks/. Accessed January 16, 2018.

Jabr F. How to really eat like a hunter–gatherer: why the Paleo diet is half-baked. *Scientific American.* June 3, 2013. https://www.scientificamerican.com/article/why-paleo-diet-half-baked-how-hunter-gatherer-really-eat/. Accessed June 9, 2017.

Lanchester J. The case against civilization: did our hunter-gatherer ancestors have it better? *New Yorker.* September 11, 2017. https://www.newyorker.com/magazine/2017/09/18/the-case-against-civilization/amp. Accessed January 16, 2017.

CHAPTER 4

Brody JE. Unlocking the secrets of the microbiome. *New York Times.* November 6, 2017. https://www.nytimes.com/2017/11/06/well/live/unlocking-the-secrets-of-the-microbiome.html. Accessed February 19, 2018.

Centers for Disease Control and Prevention. Raw milk questions and answers. How many outbreaks are related to raw milk? http://www.cdc.gov/foodsafety/rawmilk/raw-milk-questions-and-answers.html#related-outbreaks. Updated September 1, 2017. Accessed January 17, 2018.

European Food Safety Authority. The 2009 European Union report on pesticide residues in food. https://www.efsa.europa.eu/en/efsajournal/pub/2430. Published April 4, 2012. Accessed March 31, 2017.

National Academies of Sciences, Engineering, and Medicine. Board on Agriculture and Natural Resources. Genetically engineered crops: experiences and prospects. http://nas-sites.org/ge-crops/category/report/. Published May 2014. Accessed March 28, 2017.

National Institutes of Health, National Human Genome Research Institute. NIH Human Microbiome Project defines normal bacterial makeup of the body. *NIH News.* https://www.genome.gov/27549144/2012-release-nih-human-microbiome-project-defines-normal-bacterial-makeup-of-the-body/. Published June 13, 2012. Accessed February 19, 2018.

US Department of Agriculture, Economic Research Service; Martinez S, Hand MS, Da Pra M, et al. Economic research report No. ERR-97. Local food systems: concepts, impacts, and issues. https://www.ers.usda.gov/publications/pub-details/?pubid=46395. Published May 2010. Accessed March 24, 2017.

Yong E. Breast-feeding the microbiome. *New Yorker.* July 22, 2016. http://www.newyorker.com/tech/elements/breast-feeding-the-microbiome. Accessed June 28, 2017.

CHAPTER 5

Butler S. From chuck wagons to pushcarts: the history of the food truck. History.com. http://www.history.com/news/hungry-history/

from-chuck-wagons-to-pushcarts-the-history-of-the-food-truck. Published August 8, 2014. Accessed April 11, 2017.

Ferdman RA. The slow death of the home-cooked meal. *Washington Post*. March 5, 2015. https://www.washingtonpost.com/news/wonk/wp/2015/03/05/the-slow-death-of-the-home-cooked-meal/. Accessed April 10, 2017.

Food and Agriculture Organization of the United Nations. Street foods around the world. http://www.fao.org/english/newsroom/highlights/2001/010804-e.htm. Published August 21, 2001. Accessed April 11, 2017.

Gold J. How America became a food truck nation. *Smithsonian Magazine*. March 2012. http://www.smithsonianmag.com/travel/how-america-became-a-food-truck-nation-99979799/. Accessed April 11, 2017.

Okrent AM, Kumcu A. U.S. households' demand for convenience foods. US Department of Agriculture, Economic Research Service Report ERR-211. https://www.ers.usda.gov/webdocs/publications/80654/err-211.pdf?v=42668. Published July 2016. Accessed April 10, 2017.

Thompson D. Restaurants are the new factories. *Atlantic*. August 9, 2017. https://www.theatlantic.com/business/archive/2017/08/restaurant-jobs-boom/536244/. Accessed February 17, 2018.

US Department of Agriculture, Economic Research Service. Food away from home. https://www.ers.usda.gov/topics/food-choices-health/food-consumption-demand/food-away-from-home/. Updated February 8, 2018. Accessed April 10, 2017.

US National Library of Medicine. PubMed Health. How does our sense of taste work? https://www.ncbi.nlm.nih.gov/pubmedhealth/PMH0072592/. Updated August 17, 2016. Accessed May 4, 2017.

CHAPTER 6

Golden Rice Humanitarian Board. Golden Rice Project. http://www.goldenrice.org. Accessed March 5, 2018.

International Rice Research Institute. http://irri.org. Accessed March 5, 2018.

Newby PK. The future of food: how science, technology, and consumerism shape what we eat. In: Ulm W, ed. *Harvard Vision*. Cambridge, MA: Dipylon Press; 2003:3–23.

CHAPTER 7

National Institutes of Health, Office of Dietary Supplements. Vitamin D. https://ods.od.nih.gov/factsheets/VitaminD-HealthProfessional/. Updated March 2, 2018. Accessed May 13, 2017.

US Department of Agriculture, US Department of Health and Human Services. Scientific report of the 2015 Dietary Guidelines Advisory Committee. https://health.gov/dietaryguidelines/2015-scientific-report/PDFs/Scientific-Report-of-the-2015-Dietary-Guidelines-Advisory-Committee.pdf. Published February 2015. Accessed June 28, 2016.

CHAPTER 8

Amnesty International. Palm oil: global brands profiting from child and forced labour. https://www.amnesty.org/en/latest/news/2016/11/

palm-oil-global-brands-profiting-from-child-and-forced-labour/. Published November 30, 2016. Accessed February 7, 2012.

Oatman M. Stop freaking out about how much protein you're getting. *Mother Jones.* March 25, 2016. https://www.motherjones.com/environment/2016/03/your-protein-obsession-isnt-helping-anyone/. Accessed February 17, 2018.

Ranganathan J, Vennard D, Waite R, et al. Shifting diets for a sustainable food future. World Resources Institute. April 2016. http://www.wri.org/publication/shifting-diets. Accessed February 9, 2017.

Sacks MF, Lichtenstein AH, Wu JHY. Dietary fats and cardiovasular disease: a presidential advisory from the American Heart Association. *Circulation.* June 15, 2017. http://circ.ahajournals.org/content/early/2017/06/15/CIR.0000000000000510. Accessed February 6, 2017.

World Health Organization. WHO calls on countries to reduce sugars intake among adults and children. http://www.who.int/mediacentre/news/releases/2015/sugar-guideline/en/. Published March 4, 2015. Accessed May 16, 2017.

Wosen J. How coconut oil got a reputation for being healthy in the first place. *Business Insider.* June 25, 2017. http://www.businessinsider.com/how-coconut-oil-got-a-reputation-for-being-healthy-in-the-first-place-2017-6. Accessed February 6, 2018.

CHAPTER 9

American Diabetes Association. Fruits. http://www.diabetes.org/food-and-fitness/food/what-can-i-eat/making-healthy-food-choices/fruits.html. Updated December 8, 2016. Accessed June 3, 2017.

Edible seaweed. Wikipedia. https://en.wikipedia.org/wiki/Edible_seaweed. Updated February 25, 2018. Accessed March 23, 2018.

Eveleth R. There are 37.2 trillion cells in your body. *Smithsonian Magazine.* October 24, 2013. http://www.smithsonianmag.com/smart-news/there-are-372-trillion-cells-in-your-body-4941473/. Accessed August 18, 2017.

University of Delaware College of Agriculture & Natural Sciences. Using herbs and spices. http://extension.udel.edu/factsheets/using-herbs-and-spices/. Published 1914. Accessed January 23, 2018.

US Department of Agriculture, US Department of Health and Human Services. Key elements of healthy eating patterns. In: *Dietary Guidelines for Americans 2015–2020.* Washington, DC: US Department of Agriculture, US Department of Health and Human Services; 2015:chap 1. http://health.gov/dietaryguidelines/2015/guidelines/chapter-1/key-recommendations/. Published January 2016. Accessed June 27, 2016.

CHAPTER 10

Oldways Preservation Trust. Whole grain value: 2 to 3 times more of most nutrients. http://wholegrainscouncil.org/newsroom/blog/2016/06/whole-grain-value-2-to-3-times-more-of-most-nutrients. Published June 1, 2016. Accessed June 13, 2016.

Yong E. Scientists pit sourdough against white bread—with surprising results. *Atlantic.* June 6, 2017. https://www.theatlantic.com/science/archive/2017/06/sourdough-versus-white-bread/529260/?. Accessed February 20, 2018.

CHAPTER 11

Calles T. The international year of pulses: what are they and why are they important? http://www.fao.org/3/a-bl797e.pdf. Published 2016. Accessed August 14, 2017.

Togias A, Cooper SF, Acebal ML, et al. Addendum guidelines for the prevention of peanut allergy in the United States: report of the National Institute of Allergy and Infectious Diseases–sponsored expert panel. *J Allergy Clin Immunol* 2017;139(1):29–44.

CHAPTER 12

American Public Health Association. Opposition to the use of hormone growth promoters in beef and dairy cattle production. http://www.apha.org/policies-and-advocacy/public-health-policy-statements/policy-database/2014/07/09/13/42/opposition-to-the-use-of-hormone-growth-promoters-in-beef-and-dairy-cattle-production. Published November 10, 2009. Accessed July 30, 2017.

Food and Agriculture Organization of the United Nations. Greenhouse gas emissions from agriculture, forestry, and other land use. http://www.fao.org/resources/infographics/infographics-details/en/c/218650/. Published October 4, 2014. Accessed September 27, 2017.

Food and Agriculture Organization of the United Nations. Water pollution from agriculture: a global review. http://www.fao.org/3/a-i7754e.pdf. Published 2017. Accessed October 11, 2017.

Haley M. Livestock, dairy, and poultry outlook. Economic Research Service. US Department of Agriculture. https://www.ers.usda.gov/webdocs/publications/86849/ldp-m-283.pdf?v=43119. Published January 19, 2018. Accessed January 31, 2018.

Philpott T. The World Health Organization just told farmers everywhere to stop feeding antibiotics to healthy animals. *Mother Jones.* November 7, 2017. https://www.motherjones.com/food/2017/11/the-world-health-organization-just-told-farmers-everywhere-to-stop-feeding-antibiotics-to-healthy-animals/. Accessed January 28, 2018.

US Government Accountability Office. Workplace safety and health: additional data needed to address continued hazards in the meat and poultry industry. http://www.gao.gov/assets/680/676796.pdf. Published April 2016. Accessed September 18, 2017.

World Health Organization. Q & A on the carcinogenicity of the consumption of red meat and processed meat. http://www.who.int/features/qa/cancer-red-meat/en/. Published October 2015. Accessed September 29, 2017.

CHAPTER 13

American Heart Association. Fish and omega-3 fatty acids. http://www.heart.org/HEARTORG/HealthyLiving/HealthyEating/HealthyDietGoals/Fish-and-Omega-3-Fatty-Acids_UCM_303248_Article.jsp#.V5tx22ZrWo4. Published October 6, 2016. Accessed October 12, 2017.

Howard BC. Salmon farming gets leaner and greener. *National Geographic.* March 19, 2014. http://news.nationalgeographic.com/news/2014/03/140319-salmon-farming-sustainable-aquaculture/. Accessed September 29, 2017.

Institute of Medicine. *Seafood Choices: Balancing Benefits and Risks*. https://
www.nap.edu/catalog/11762/seafood-choices-balancing-benefits-and-risks.
Washington, DC: National Academies Press; 2007. Accessed September
20, 2017.

Lawrence F. If consumers knew how farmed chickens were raised, they
might never eat their meat again. *Guardian*. April 24, 2016. https://www.
theguardian.com/environment/2016/apr/24/real-cost-of-roast-chicken-
animal-welfare-farms. Accessed January 30, 2018.

Lazar A. Better practices: A market transformed. *WWF Magazine*. Fall 2014.
https://www.worldwildlife.org/magazine/issues/fall-2014/articles/better-
practices-a-market-transformed. Accessed September 29, 2017.

US Food & Drug Administration. Eating fish: what pregnant woman and
parents should know. https://www.fda.gov/Food/ResourcesForYou/
Consumers/ucm393070.htm. Published August 8, 2017. Accessed October
12, 2017.

Vidal J. Salmon farming in crisis: 'We are seeing a chemical arms race in the seas.'
Guardian. April 1, 2017. https://www.theguardian.com/environment/2017/
apr/01/is-farming-salmon-bad-for-the-environment. Accessed October 12,
2017.

CHAPTER 14

American Dental Association. Fluoride in water. http://www.ada.org/en/public-
programs/advocating-for-the-public/fluoride-and-fluoridation. Accessed May
29, 2017.

Charles D. Coffee for a cause: what do those feel-good labels deliver? *NPR Morning
Edition*. April 24, 2013. http://www.npr.org/sections/thesalt/2013/04/
24/177757797/coffee-for-a-cause-what-do-those-feel-good-labels-deliver.
Accessed July 6, 2017.

Nace T. We're now at a million plastic bottles per minute—91% of which are not
recycled. *Forbes*. July 26, 2017. https://www.forbes.com/sites/trevornace/
2017/07/26/million-plastic-bottles-minute-91-not-recycled/#341c3864292c.
Accessed March 7, 2018.

PubMed Health. Does coffee make you live longer? https://www.ncbi.nlm.nih.
gov/pubmedhealth/behindtheheadlines/news/2017-07-12-does-coffee-make-
you-live-longer/. Published July 12, 2017. Accessed February 19, 2018.

Schlossberg T. Bottled water or tap: how much does your choice matter?
New York Times. October 20, 2016. https://www.nytimes.com/interactive/
2016/science/bottled-water-or-tap.html. Accessed March 7, 2018.

CHAPTER 15

LoConte NK, Brewster AM, Kaur JS, et al. Alcohol and cancer: a statement of the
American Society of Clinical Oncology. *J Clin Oncol*. 2018;36(1):83–93.

CHAPTER 16

Byrd-Bredbenner C, Ferruzzi MG, Fulgoni VL 3rd, et al. Satisfying America's fruit
gap: summary of an expert roundtable on the role of 100% fruit juice. *J Food
Sci*. 2017;82:1523–1534.

Center for Science in the Public Interest. Soda companies turning to low- and middle-income countries to replace sagging U.S. sales. https://cspinet.org/new/201602091.html. Published February 9, 2016. Accessed March 7, 2018.

Watson K, Treanor S. The Mexicans dying for a fizzy drink. *BBC News.* http://www.bbc.com/news/magazine-35461270. Published February 2, 2016. Accessed March 7, 2018.

CHAPTER 17

Best diets overall. *U.S. News & World Report.* http://health.usnews.com/best-diet/best-diets-overall. Published 2017. Accessed October 20, 2017.

Calerie. https://calerie.duke.edu. Accessed October 20, 2017.

Food and Agriculture Organization of the United Nations. Food-based dietary guidelines. Dietary guidelines and sustainability. http://www.fao.org/nutrition/education/food-dietary-guidelines/background/sustainable-dietary-guidelines/en/. Accessed November 10, 2017.

Friend T. Silicon Valley's quest to live forever. *New Yorker.* April 3, 2017. https://www.newyorker.com/magazine/2017/04/03/silicon-valleys-quest-to-live-forever. Accessed February 20, 2018.

National Institute of Nutrition. *Dietary Guidelines for Indians: A Manual.* 2nd ed. Hyderabad, India: National Institute of Nutrition; 2011. http://ninindia.org/dietaryguidelinesforninwebsite.pdf. Accessed October 24 2017.

NHS Choices. The Eatwell Guide. https://www.nhs.uk/Livewell/Goodfood/Pages/the-eatwell-guide.aspx. Updated March 16, 2016. Accessed October 23, 2017.

Rangathan J, Waite R. Sustainable diets: what you need to know in 12 charts. World Resources Institute. http://www.wri.org/blog/2016/04/sustainable-diets-what-you-need-know-12-charts. Published April 20, 2016. Accessed November 18, 2017.

US Department of Health and Human Services, US Department of Agriculture. *Dietary Guidelines for Americans 2015–2020.* 8th ed. Washington, DC: US Department of Health and Human Services, US Department of Agriculture; 2015. https://health.gov/dietaryguidelines/2015/guidelines/. Published January 2016. Accessed October 23, 2017.

World Health Organization. Global strategy on diet, physical activity and health. http://www.who.int/dietphysicalactivity/diet-overview/en/. Accessed October 24, 2017.

WorldWatch Institute. Is meat sustainable? http://www.worldwatch.org/node/549. Accessed November 11, 2017.

CHAPTER 18

Brodwin E. This Cornell scientist saved an $11-million industry—and ignited the GMO wars. *Business Insider.* June 23, 2017. http://www.businessinsider.com/gmo-controversy-beginning-fruit-2017-6. Accessed December 18, 2017.

Chen T-P. In China, a robot's place is in the kitchen. *Wall Street Journal.* July 24, 2016. https://www.wsj.com/articles/in-china-a-robots-place-is-in-the-kitchen-1469393604. Accessed December 30, 2017.

Davis N, Burgen S, Corbyn Z. Future of food: how we cook. *Guardian.* September 13, 2015. https://www.theguardian.com/technology/2015/sep/13/future-of-food-how-we-cook. Accessed December 30, 2017.

Ekekwe N. How digital farming is changing farming in Africa. *Harvard Business Review.* May 18, 2017. https://hbr.org/2017/05/how-digital-technology-is-changing-farming-in-africa/. Accessed December 31, 2017.

Estes AC. 13 fascinating farming robots that will feed humans of the future. *Gizmodo.* http://gizmodo.com/13-fascinating-farming-robots-that-will-feed-our-future-1683489468. Published February 3, 2015. Accessed December 16, 2017.

European Parliamentary Research Service. Precision agriculture and the future of farming in Europe. December, 2016. www.europarl.europa.eu/RegData/etudes/STUD/2016/581892/EPRS_STU(2016)581892_EN.pdf. Accessed December 18, 2017.

Fleming A. Could lab-grown fish and meat feed the world—without killing a single animal? *Guardian.* September 20, 2017. https://www.theguardian.com/lifeandstyle/2017/sep/20/lab-grown-meat-fish-feed-the-world-frankenmeat-startups. Accessed December 20, 2017.

Food and Agriculture Organization of the United Nations. Sustainable development goals. http://www.fao.org/sustainable-development-goals/en/. Published January 2016. Accessed December 31, 2017.

Food and Agriculture Organization of the United Nations. The future of food and agriculture: trends and challenges. http://www.fao.org/3/a-i6583e.pdf. Published 2017. Accessed December 18, 2017.

Frazier I. The vertical farm. *New Yorker.* January 9, 2017. https://www.newyorker.com/magazine/2017/01/09/the-vertical-farm. Accessed December 20, 2017.

Gamble J. Soylent is healthier than the average North American diet. *Atlantic.* July 11, 2016. https://www.theatlantic.com/health/archive/2016/07/soylent-is-healthier-than-our-diet/489830/. Accessed December 31, 2017.

Mwesigwa A. Can a GM banana solve Uganda's hunger crisis? *Guardian.* December 12, 2017. https://www.theguardian.com/global-development/2017/dec/12/gm-genetically-modified-banana-uganda-hunger-crisis. Accessed December 18, 2017.

Patil A. How the Internet of Things can completely redefine your kitchen. *IoT Global Network.* http://www.iotglobalnetwork.com/iotdir/2017/06/08/how-the-internet-of-things-can-completely-redefine-your-kitchen-6006/. Published June 8, 2017. Accessed December 31, 2017.

The complete list of references can be downloaded from pknewby.com.

INDEX